NEW FR~~ ~~ IN CONTRACEPTIVE RESEARCH

A Blueprint for Action

Sharyl J. Nass and Jerome F. Strauss III, *Editors*

Committee on New Frontiers in Contraceptive Research
Board on Health Sciences Policy

INSTITUTE OF MEDICINE
OF THE NATIONAL ACADEMIES

THE NATIONAL ACADEMIES PRESS
Washington, D.C.
www.nap.edu

THE NATIONAL ACADEMIES PRESS   500 FIFTH STREET, N.W.   Washington, DC 20001

NOTICE: The project that is the subject of this report was approved by the Governing Board of the National Research Council, whose members are drawn from the councils of the National Academy of Sciences, the National Academy of Engineering, and the Institute of Medicine. The members of the committee responsible for the report were chosen for their special competences and with regard for appropriate balance.

Support for this project was provided by the Bill and Melinda Gates Foundation. The views presented in this report are those of the Institute of Medicine Committee on New Frontiers in Contraceptive Research and are not necessarily those of the funding agency.

Library of Congress Cataloging-in-Publication Data

New frontiers in contraceptive research : a blueprint for action / Sharyl J. Nass and Jerome F. Strauss III, editors ; Committee on New Frontiers in Contraceptive Research, Board on Health Sciences Policy.
        p. ; cm.
    Includes bibliographical references.
    ISBN 0-309-09107-1 (pbk.)
    1. Contraception—Research.
    [DNLM: 1. Contraception—methods. WP 630 N5324 2003] I. Nass, Sharyl J. II. Strauss, Jerome F. (Jerome Frank), 1947- III. Institute of Medicine (U.S.). Committee on New Frontiers in Contraceptive Research.
    RG136.N493 2003
    613.9′4′072—dc22
                                2003027272

Additional copies of this report are available from the National Academies Press, 500 Fifth Street, N.W., Lockbox 285, Washington, DC 20055; (800) 624-6242 or (202) 334-3313 (in the Washington metropolitan area); Internet, http://www.nap.edu.

For more information about the Institute of Medicine, visit the IOM home page at: **www.iom.edu.**

Copyright 2004 by the National Academy of Sciences. All rights reserved.

Printed in the United States of America.

The serpent has been a symbol of long life, healing, and knowledge among almost all cultures and religions since the beginning of recorded history. The serpent adopted as a logotype by the Institute of Medicine is a relief carving from ancient Greece, now held by the Staatliche Museen in Berlin.

"Knowing is not enough; we must apply.
Willing is not enough; we must do."
—Goethe

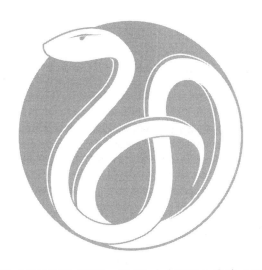

INSTITUTE OF MEDICINE
OF THE NATIONAL ACADEMIES

Shaping the Future for Health

THE NATIONAL ACADEMIES
Advisers to the Nation on Science, Engineering, and Medicine

The **National Academy of Sciences** is a private, nonprofit, self-perpetuating society of distinguished scholars engaged in scientific and engineering research, dedicated to the furtherance of science and technology and to their use for the general welfare. Upon the authority of the charter granted to it by the Congress in 1863, the Academy has a mandate that requires it to advise the federal government on scientific and technical matters. Dr. Bruce M. Alberts is president of the National Academy of Sciences.

The **National Academy of Engineering** was established in 1964, under the charter of the National Academy of Sciences, as a parallel organization of outstanding engineers. It is autonomous in its administration and in the selection of its members, sharing with the National Academy of Sciences the responsibility for advising the federal government. The National Academy of Engineering also sponsors engineering programs aimed at meeting national needs, encourages education and research, and recognizes the superior achievements of engineers. Dr. Wm. A. Wulf is president of the National Academy of Engineering.

The **Institute of Medicine** was established in 1970 by the National Academy of Sciences to secure the services of eminent members of appropriate professions in the examination of policy matters pertaining to the health of the public. The Institute acts under the responsibility given to the National Academy of Sciences by its congressional charter to be an adviser to the federal government and, upon its own initiative, to identify issues of medical care, research, and education. Dr. Harvey V. Fineberg is president of the Institute of Medicine.

The **National Research Council** was organized by the National Academy of Sciences in 1916 to associate the broad community of science and technology with the Academy's purposes of furthering knowledge and advising the federal government. Functioning in accordance with general policies determined by the Academy, the Council has become the principal operating agency of both the National Academy of Sciences and the National Academy of Engineering in providing services to the government, the public, and the scientific and engineering communities. The Council is administered jointly by both Academies and the Institute of Medicine. Dr. Bruce M. Alberts and Dr. Wm. A. Wulf are chair and vice chair, respectively, of the National Research Council.

www.national-academies.org

COMMITTEE ON NEW FRONTIERS IN CONTRACEPTIVE RESEARCH

JEROME F. STRAUSS III, M.D., Ph.D. (*Chair*), The Luigi Mastroianni, Jr. Professor and Director, Center for Research on Reproduction and Women's Health, University of Pennsylvania Medical Center; Philadelphia, PA

LISA BRANNON-PEPPAS, M.S., Ph.D., Research Professor, The University of Texas at Austin, Austin, TX

ROBERT E. BRAUN, Ph.D., Associate Professor, University of Washington, Seattle, WA

MARLENE L. COHEN, Ph.D., Vice President, Creative Pharmacology Solutions, LLC, Carmel, IN

VANESSA E. CULLINS, M.D., M.P.H., M.B.A., Vice President of Medical Affairs, Planned Parenthood Federation of America, New York, NY

JACQUELINE E. DARROCH, Ph.D., Senior Vice President, Vice President for Science, The Alan Guttmacher Institute, New York, NY

MAHMOUD FATHALLA, M.D., Professor of Obstetrics and Gynecology, Assiut University, Assiut, Egypt

LINDA C. GIUDICE, M.D., Ph.D., Professor, Director, Division of Reproductive Endocrinology and Infertility, and Director, Women's Health at Stanford, Department of Gynecology and Obstetrics, Stanford University Medical Center, Stanford, CA

ANNA GLASIER, M.D., Director of Family Planning Services, Lothian Primary Care Trust, and University of Edinburgh, Edinburgh, Scotland

MICHAEL HARPER, Ph.D., Sc.D., M.B.A., Professor, Department of Obstetrics and Gynecology, Eastern Virginia Medical School, and Director of CICCR and GMP, CONRAD, Arlington, VA

GREGORY S. KOPF, Ph.D., Assistant Vice President, Discovery Women's Health Research Institute, Wyeth Research, Collegeville, PA

MARTIN M. MATZUK, M.D., Ph.D., Stuart A. Wallace Chair and Professor, Departments of Pathology, Molecular and Cellular Biology, and Molecular and Human Genetics, Baylor College of Medicine, Houston, TX

RUTH MERKATZ, R.N., Ph.D., Director of Women's Health, Pfizer Inc, New York, NY

NANCY PADIAN, M.P.H., Ph.D., Professor, Department of Obstetrics, Gynecology and Reproductive Sciences, and Director of Women's Global Health Imperative and of International Research, AIDS Research Institute, University of California, San Francisco, San Francisco, CA

REGINE L. SITRUK-WARE, M.D., Executive Director, Product Research and Development, Center for Biomedical Research, Population Council, New York, NY

STUDY STAFF

SHARYL J. NASS, Ph.D., Study Director
JANICE MEHLER, Visiting Staff Officer
MARYJOY BALLANTYNE, Research Associate (through August 2003)
SHIRA H. FISCHER, Research Assistant (from July 2003)
NAKIA JOHNSON, Senior Project Assistant

DIVISION STAFF

ANDREW POPE, Ph.D., Director, Board on Health Sciences Policy
TROY PRINCE, Administrative Assistant
CARLOS GABRIEL, Financial Associate

Reviewers

This report has been reviewed in draft form by individuals chosen for their diverse perspectives and technical expertise, in accordance with procedures approved by the NRC's Report Review Committee. The purpose of this independent review is to provide candid and critical comments that will assist the institution in making its published report as sound as possible and to ensure that the report meets institutional standards for objectivity, evidence, and responsiveness to the study charge. The review comments and draft manuscript remain confidential to protect the integrity of the deliberative process. We wish to thank the following individuals for their review of this report:

STEVEN J. BRICKNER, Pfizer, Inc
WILLARD CATES, Family Health International
MITCHELL CREININ, University of Pittsburgh, Magee-Womens
    Hospital
JURRIEN DEAN, National Institutes of Health
GORDON W. DUNCAN, Consultant, Seattle, WA
ELLEN HARDY, State University of Campinas, Brazil
BARRY T. HINTON, The University of Virginia
JANE MENKEN, University of Colorado
LISA RARICK, Reproductive Health and Regulatory Affairs
    Consultant, Gaithersburg, MD
HENRY W. RIECKEN, University of Pennsylvania, Retired

Although the reviewers listed above have provided many constructive comments and suggestions, they were not asked to endorse the conclusions or recommendations nor did they see the final draft of the report before its release. The review of this report was overseen by **Mary Lake Polan**, Stanford University School of Medicine, and by **Mary Jane Osborn**, University of Connecticut Health Center. Appointed by the National Research Council and Institute of Medicine, they were responsible for making certain that an independent examination of this report was carried out in accordance with institutional procedures and that all review comments were carefully considered. Responsibility for the final content of this report rests entirely with the authoring committee and the institution.

Preface

The Institute of Medicine (IOM) began producing reports on contraceptive development in 1989 and its most recent report, *Contraceptive Research and Development: Looking to the Future*, was issued in 1996. Why is another report on contraception needed at this time?

As the committee documents in this report, unintended pregnancy remains a major problem. Recent survey data are very consistent: more than a quarter of pregnancies worldwide are unintended. Moreover, between 1995 and 2000 nearly 700,000 women died and many more experienced illness, injury, and disability as a result of unplanned pregnancy. Even in cases in which maternal health is maintained, an unintended pregnancy can cause significant harm for families and communities—emotional, social, and economic. Dual protection from pregnancy and HIV/AIDS infection remains elusive, while the pandemic of HIV/AIDS continues to devastate sub-Saharan Africa and Southeast Asia. The cost of contraceptive products and the availability and adoption of existing contraceptive methods still remain challenges to international family planning efforts. At the same time there is increasing recognition that a wider range of modalities is needed to address the changing contraceptive needs of the populations of the world across the reproductive life cycle. This unmet need has not been a major priority of the research community and pharmaceutical industry.

Since the release of the last IOM report, there has been a remarkable scientific revolution. The human genome has been sequenced, and many new technologies that can be used to study biological systems on an unprecedented scale are now available. As a result, the opportunities to identify novel targets for contraceptives are extraordinary. Advances in materials science, drug development, and drug delivery may also facilitate the introduction of new and innovative contraceptive methods. Thus, the time is right for a reevaluation of the research agenda in the field.

Unfortunately, at this time of opportunity, there is flagging interest in contraceptive development, not only in the pharmaceutical industry but also in the academic scientific community. There are a number of factors which have contributed to this, including the obstacles to contraceptive development that were identified in the past reports, particularly the 1996 report, which continue to challenge the field. However, new paradigms for science have emerged in the past few years, including large-scale collaborative science and new vehicles for public–private collaboration. New parties are also interested in the process of contraceptive development and dissemination, and new global consortia are dealing with reproductive health.

Science, product development, and implementation are all addressed in the recommendations developed by the committee. Although contraceptive research, development, and use in the United States and abroad are influenced by political context, the committee restricted its deliberations to scientific issues and ways in which science could best address global concerns of fertility regulation and reproductive health. It is not possible to predict which of the specific recommendations are likely to yield the greatest benefits. Indeed, although our recommendations are diverse, all are interconnected and important for improving the range of products, their efficacies, and their acceptability. It is the committee's hope that sponsors, both public and private, will find topics of interest among this menu of research goals.

The committee chose not to estimate the costs of implementing the research agenda. Costs will vary depending on the scale, scope, and time frame of a given research program, and costs will change as science and technology progress. Certainly, completing the research agenda outlined here will require significant financial resources, but given the unmet needs and the unprecedented opportunities before us, the time seems right to launch a broad and ambitious initiative. Traditionally, much of the federal investment in biomedical research has focused on treating and curing diseases, many of which primarily affect individuals at a late stage of life. The development of novel contraceptives, in contrast, offers a cost-effective preventive approach that could improve the health, quality of life, and longevity of millions of people worldwide, particularly young adults and their children.

On behalf of the committee, I thank the Bill and Melinda Gates Foundation for its generous support of this study and for its vision of a world made better by the availability of more effective contraception. The committee itself was, without exception, involved, constructive, and hard working. We came from many different perspectives—biological sciences, medicine, product development, social sciences, and service delivery—yet we forged a common understanding of how to achieve our shared goal of improving the lives of families worldwide. I thank the members for their individual contributions and for their collective accomplishments.

The committee owes a debt of gratitude to the IOM staff. Sharyl Nass, as study director, was a full intellectual participant in the study and the guiding spirit in writing the report. It is because of her skillful project management and writing abilities that this project was completed successfully and swiftly. MaryJoy Ballantyne and, later, Shira Fischer, provided excellent and dedicated research support, and were instrumental in maintaining the study timetable. Nakia Johnson handled the logistics of our meetings, international conference, and report production. Janice Mehler, on loan to the committee from the National Academies' Report Review Committee, not only provided insight into the review process but also contributed invaluable assistance with the research and writing. Steven Marcus produced a written summary of the workshop proceedings, and Michael Hayes served as copy editor of the report.

We are also indebted to the many participants in the workshop that we held on July 15-16, 2003. The ideas expressed by the speakers and attendees were a fundamental contribution to this report. The workshop agenda, speakers, and attendees are provided in Appendix B.

Finally, I wish to acknowledge other individuals who provided valuable input to the committee, verbally or in written form, during the course of the study, including David Archer, Diana Blithe, Doug Colvard, Mitchell Creinin, Carl Djerassi, Florence Haseltine, Joanne Luoto, Kate Moore, Susan Newcomer, Paolo Rinaudo, Robert Spirtas, Michael Thomas, Kirsten Vogelsong, Livia Wan, and James Wootton.

In 1965, Gregory Pincus wrote that his interest in fertility regulation was stimulated primarily by Mrs. Margaret Sanger, who visited him and expressed the hope that a relatively simple and foolproof method of contraception might be developed through laboratory research. The result of that visit was research that led to the development of the oral contraceptive pill. This vision of how science can serve humanity should continue to guide us in the development of the next generation of contraceptive products.

Jerome F. Strauss III
Chair

Contents

xiii

NEW FRONTIERS
IN CONTRACEPTIVE
RESEARCH

Executive Summary

THE NEED FOR NEW CONTRACEPTIVES

Family planning is a socially beneficial activity that affects the well-being of women, men, children, families, and society as a whole. Planned fertility confers the benefits of improved child health and development through the more effective intergenerational transfer of resources and the increased longevity and empowerment of women, with its attendant economic benefits to the family and the community. It reduces the lifetime risk of chronic illness or death from a pregnancy-related condition. Barrier methods of contraception have the added benefit of lessening the likelihood of transmission of sexually transmitted infections (STIs).

Conversely, a woman experiencing an unintended pregnancy is at greater risk for depression and physical abuse. She also faces the usual health risks of pregnancy, including maternal death. Closely spaced births carry additional health risks for the mother and child. The child born from an unplanned conception is at greater risk of low birth weight, of dying in its first year of life, of being abused, and of not receiving sufficient resources for healthy development. With an unplanned conception, the mother and father may suffer economic hardship and may fail to achieve their educational and career goals, and their relationship is at greater risk of dissolution.

According to a recent analysis by the Global Health Council, the world's 1.3 billion women between the ages of 15 and 45 experienced more than 1.2 billion pregnancies in the 6 years between 1995 and 2000 (Global Health Council, 2002). Of these, more than 300 million—or more than one-

1

quarter—were unintended, and nearly 700,000 women died as a result of unintended pregnancies. The number of women at risk for unplanned pregnancies will grow as the world's population continues to rise. Over the next decade, 600 million girls are projected to reach adolescence, which will be the largest cohort of young women in human history.

Although a number of reversible and nonreversible contraceptive methods are generally effective (barrier methods, hormonal methods, intrauterine devices, and contraceptive sterilization), no method is 100 percent effective for all users, and some men and women experience undesirable side effects. Studies have shown that more than 120 million women around the world report that they are sexually active, do not want to become pregnant, and are not using any form of contraception whether because of cost, governmental policy, lack of access, or other reasons.

Most men and women spend the majority of their reproductive years trying to avoid conception, and their contraceptive preferences change during the 30 years that they typically need contraception. Methods are needed for child spacing as well as permanent pregnancy prevention, for young people and those approaching menopause, and for postpartum and breast-feeding women. Methods are also needed for women and men with medical conditions that restrict contraceptive options, for those with few resources, for those with limited access to medical care, and for those whose personal situations make correct and consistent use difficult. The cultural or personal unacceptability of the various methods also points to the need for new options. In addition, the development of new methods that protect against pregnancy as well as against STIs would be enormously beneficial, as the HIV/AIDS pandemic threatens world health and continues to devastate sub-Saharan Africa and Asia.

Recent scientific and technological advances in genomics, proteomics, new materials, and new drug delivery systems, along with a new understanding of reproductive biology offer the promise of new, safe, and effective forms of contraception. At the same time, new global consortia working in this area are beginning to provide improved structures to pursue these opportunities collaboratively. The development of novel contraceptives would help alleviate the growing unmet demand for satisfactory contraception and would improve the lives of families everywhere. Given the unprecedented opportunities for new progress in the field, now is the time to move forward with a bold research agenda.

ABOUT THIS REPORT

At the request of the Bill and Melinda Gates Foundation, the Institute of Medicine (IOM) established the Committee on New Frontiers in Contraceptive Research to explore scientific opportunities for improving contraceptives. The committee was asked to organize an international symposium that brought together individuals with expertise in contraception, basic reproductive biology, new technologies, product development, behavioral science, and international health. The objective was to bring new concepts and analytical frameworks to the discussion of contraceptive research and development. Following the symposium, the committee deliberated on the important issues that were raised at the workshop, in the literature, and from their own experiences. On the basis of those discussions, the committee was charged with producing this report, which identifies priority areas for future research and development in the field of contraception.

This report builds on *Contraceptive Research and Development: Looking to the Future* (Institute of Medicine, 1996), the most recent of several IOM reports about the future of contraceptive research and development. Many of the recommendations put forth in that report are as relevant today as they were in 1996, but the recent unprecedented advances in science and technology warrant a fresh examination of the research goals and agenda in the field of contraception. Although progress has been made since that report was released in 1996, the contraceptive modalities recently developed or introduced are based mainly on preexisting technologies and approaches. The progress in some areas thought to be promising in 1996 has been minimal, and recent discoveries provide new perspectives on previously recommended targets. A major goal of the present committee was to identify ways in which new information and new technologies can be rapidly and efficiently applied to contraceptive target identification, validation, and product development. Moreover, the committee found that there is still a great need to reenergize the field and to translate significant observations from the science of reproductive biology to practical applications in fertility regulation.

The committee's recommendations, summarized in the following sections and in Box ES-1, address (1) facilitation of the stages of contraceptive development from target selection to product development and clinical testing and (2) strategies for research success, including participation by developing countries, expansion of public–private partnerships, increased clinical and scientific training and career development in contraception, and strategic management of research efforts. These recommendations cover a diverse range of topics, but all are interconnected and important for improving the range of available contraceptive products, their efficacies, and their acceptabilities.

BOX ES-1
Summary of Recommendations: A Blueprint for Action

Recommendations

Identify and Validate Novel Contraceptive Targets (Chapter 2)
1. Generate a complete reproductive transcriptome and proteome, and define genetic and protein networks.
2. Generate reproductive lipidomes and glycomes.
3. Validate existing and emerging contraceptive targets.

Enhance Contraceptive Drug Discovery, Development, and Clinical Testing (Chapters 3 and 4)
4. Develop high-throughput screening facilities.
5. Facilitate translational research.
6. Facilitate the development of appropriate drug delivery systems.
7. Develop new approaches to measure contraceptive efficacy.
8. Integrate behavioral research at an early stage of development.
9. Discover, enhance, and promote potential health benefits of existing and new methods, and intensify efforts to develop new contraceptive methods that are prophylactic for HIV infection and other STIs.

Facilitate and Coordinate Future Implementation of Contraceptive Research and Development (Chapter 5)
10. Expand public–private partnerships for contraceptive development.
11. Increase the participation of developing countries in contraceptive development.
12. Increase training and career development opportunities in contraception.
13. Establish an ongoing Forum on Contraceptive Research and Development and create an Alliance for Contraceptive Development.

FROM TARGET SELECTION TO PRODUCT DEVELOPMENT

Identify and Validate Novel Contraceptive Targets

In the course of genomics research, thousands of genes expressed in the reproductive cells and tissues of model organisms and humans have been identified, and many of these sequences appear to be unique to reproductive tissues and gametes. Remarkably, a recent study found that 4 percent of all genes may be uniquely and exclusively expressed in male germ cells. More than 200 human genes or related genes in other species have been shown genetically to play roles in reproduction in vivo. Recent research in proteomics has also led to the discovery of proteins that are unique to reproductive cells and tissues. The identification of genes and proteins that are expressed specifically in the reproductive tract and, more importantly, that function specifically in the reproductive tract could lead to the development of new contraceptives that specifically affect the reproductive tract and thus produce minimal unwanted side effects.

More work is needed to define more completely those genes and proteins that are unique to reproductive tissues and that are essential for reproductive function. Knowledge about how genes and proteins interact to form regulatory networks will also be important for the identification of key molecular targets for contraceptive development. In addition, more information about the structures and functions of the lipid and carbohydrate components of reproductive tissues could lead to the development of new contraceptive approaches.

Recommendation 1: Identify and characterize all genes and proteins uniquely or preferentially expressed in the testis, ovary, and reproductive tissues; and define the genetic and protein networks in cells relevant to reproduction, including construction of a protein interaction map for the sperm and the egg.

- Develop and apply selective screening methods to identify classes of molecules that have been traditionally targeted by pharmaceuticals, including membrane proteins, enzymes, receptors, and ion channels and transporter proteins.
- Continue the funding of research in progress to define the reproductive transcriptome.
- Convene a broad group of reproductive biologists, bioinformaticists, biochemists, and physiologists to verify, annotate, and standardize all gene expression data obtained by genomic methods. The information generated should then be stored in readily accessible databases based on the World Wide Web.
- Determine the complete proteomes of the sperm and the egg.
- Immediately initiate long-term support for efforts to identify and construct regulatory networks in reproductive cells, since genes and proteins do not act autonomously.

Recommendation 2: Generate lipidomes and glycomes of the reproductive tract tissues and mature gametes.

- Determine the unique carbohydrate structures on proteins and lipids in reproductive tract cells.

- Determine the contents and organizations of lipid domains within the membranes of reproductive tract cells.
- Determine the roles of carbohydrates and lipids in reproductive tract cells to identify targets for small molecules that could act selectively to disrupt membrane structure and function.

Recommendation 3: Validate existing and emerging contraceptive targets by using forward and reverse genetic approaches with model organisms.

- Make use of existing genetic models through more in-depth phenotypic analysis. This includes characterization by both genomic (e.g., microarray screening) and proteomic (e.g., global changes in protein modification) methods.
- Fund a small consortium of investigators (public or private) for the sole purpose of completing the genetic validation of all potential targets. Ideally, conditional gene knockout approaches should be used to reduce expression in specific adult tissues in order to replicate the use of contraceptives and to avoid artifacts due to developmental defects.
- Newly established genetic models should be rapidly distributed to the community of scientists involved in reproductive biology research for prompt and comprehensive phenotypic analysis.

Accelerate the Discovery and Development of Compounds That Modulate Existing and Emerging Targets

Several promising new targets for contraceptive development have already been identified, and many more will undoubtedly be discovered through efforts to implement Recommendations 1 to 3. However, validated targets are useful only if compounds can be identified to modulate those targets in humans, and it remains a challenge to select lead molecules for drug development. The most efficient way to initially identify such compounds is by using high-throughput drug discovery approaches. The effort will also require a variety of experimental approaches, from in vitro studies to whole-animal studies, to evaluate lead molecules for the purpose of subsequent clinical development (translational research). Much of the basic research that can lead to the discovery of potential drug targets is undertaken in university laboratories, but university-based researchers have inadequate access to the resources and information needed to develop compounds for the most promising targets that they have identified, and they lack access to the large, diverse libraries of compounds for screening as found in the pharmaceutical sector.

Recommendation 4: Implement a mechanism and infrastructure for high-throughput screening facilities and the development of international chemical libraries.

- Support two to four not-for-profit institutions with data-sharing capacities to develop high-throughput screening facilities for public use.
- Support and maintain two to four publicly accessible chemical libraries useful for drug development (i.e., via the elimination of potentially toxic molecules, metabolically active molecules, etc.) in not-for-profit organizations. The establishment of a "bioactive small-molecule library," as recently outlined in the National Institutes of Health (NIH) Roadmap,[1] could potentially meet this goal, depending on how that program is structured.
- Seek advice from the legal community regarding intellectual property ownership as it pertains to such a shared infrastructure for compound screening and chemical library development.
- Apply high-throughput drug discovery technologies to promising contraceptive target molecules or processes (as they are discovered and for those that have already been identified).
- Identify specific compounds that could be exploited as new contraceptives with noncontraceptive health benefits (e.g., compounds with both contraceptive and antimicrobial properties).
- Develop information technology that can be used internationally to facilitate sharing of and public access to high-throughput screening and chemical libraries.

Recommendation 5: Implement mechanisms to accelerate contraceptive product development and clinical testing once a lead molecule or concept prototype has been discovered in an academic laboratory by sharing multidisciplinary national and international resources. Specifically:

- Create a special projects program in NIH, affiliated with the Contraceptive Clinical Trials network, to fund the development of novel contraceptive compounds that offer large potential benefits for the global community. Such a program could perhaps be modeled after the National Cancer Institute's Rapid Access to Intervention Development program, designed to assist with the clinical translation of new therapeutics that have been discovered in the academic community but for which there is limited interest or capacity for further development in the private sector.

---

[1]See www.nihroadmap.nih.gov (accessed October 2003).

- Provide incentives to the pharmaceutical and biotechnology industries to expand their contraceptive research and development programs and their collaborative interactions with the public sector to develop contraceptives that meet the needs of populations in both developed and developing countries.
- Provide adequate funding for contract laboratories to partner with the public sector to make materials, test the compositions of lead molecules, and evaluate the pharmacokinetic and toxicological properties of lead molecules.
- Support existing not-for-profit infrastructures and promote and fund the development of consortia to perform translational activities for basic researchers.

Apply Recent Advances in Drug Delivery Systems

Delivery systems for contraceptive agents to date have focused on oral, transdermal, subcutaneous, intrauterine, and vaginal delivery modalities of small molecules. With the advent of the genomic and proteomic revolutions, alternative delivery systems will be necessary to accommodate new generations of contraceptives in a cost-effective manner. The particular delivery mode that is ultimately selected depends on multiple factors, including the physiochemical properties and metabolic stability of the compound, the target, and user acceptability. The science of drug delivery systems is constantly evolving and is technically demanding, highly specialized, and costly. Although most pharmaceutical companies have dedicated groups with expertise in delivery systems, only a few investigators outside of the pharmaceutical industry specialize in this particular applied science. This limits the ability of investigators in not-for-profit organizations to use these technologies in the development of their compounds.

Recommendation 6: Develop mechanisms to access, apply, and enhance the technology of drug delivery and formulation science to contraceptive development.

- Consider and select the best formulation and delivery system for each compound at an early stage of development, with consideration given to the physiochemical properties of the compound, the target, and user acceptability. One possible approach is to establish consulting programs in drug formulation and delivery systems available to scientists requiring this expertise.
- Develop new delivery systems for compounds with unique physiochemical properties (e.g., peptides) and to enable the specific and

local delivery of existing and new compounds to a target in the reproductive tract.

Accelerate and Improve Clinical Testing of New Contraceptive Methods

New methods of contraception must offer high levels of effectiveness if they are to be approved by the drug regulatory authorities and if they are to meet user needs. However, measuring effectiveness is not easy. For both ethical and practical reasons, phase I and many phase II clinical trials typically do not use pregnancy as the end point but rather use a surrogate marker of fertility, such as ovulation or sperm count. The assessment of such markers involves the use of expensive tests, which require skilled investigators and which make huge demands on the time and goodwill of the participants. The capacity of each marker to accurately reflect sterility varies, and the contraceptive method dictates which markers can be used. The choice of surrogate markers of sterility may be even more challenging for some of the future potential methods of contraception because they will likely target completely new pathways or steps in reproduction. Researchers can benefit from dialogue with regulatory bodies to address the unique aspects of contraceptive development and to design new approaches to clinical trials.

Recommendation 7: Develop new approaches to measure contraceptive efficacy that can reduce the time from phase I and II trials to large-scale clinical testing.

- Develop new surrogate markers to measure sterility, including those relevant for novel contraceptive targets.
- Develop acceptable new study designs for clinical trials of contraceptives.

Consider Usability Early in Development

To be successful, contraceptive methods must be attractive to potential users and must be feasible for distribution systems to provide. If either of these is likely to be an impediment, it would be best to know that before investing a large effort into product development and clinical trials. There are a number of options for integrating behavioral and operations research into or in parallel with early stage clinical studies so that they will be complementary to the efficient measurement of safety and efficacy.

Recommendation 8: Provide incentives and mechanisms for the integration of behavioral and operations research, including the views of providers as well as those of potential users and their partners, early in the contraceptive research and development process.

- Develop tools that can more accurately measure acceptability and potential use, and can more accurately predict the characteristics of contraceptive methods that will be attractive to users in different settings and life stages.
- Determine which service delivery practices are effective in improving provider and consumer acceptance and use of contraceptive methods.

Develop Contraceptive Methods with Other Benefits

Most couples need to use contraception for roughly 30 years simply for pregnancy prevention. Health benefits beyond pregnancy prevention offer significant added value to long-term users of a particular contraceptive method who tolerate the method solely for its contraceptive benefit. Benefits of current methods include alleviation of dysmenorrhea, acne, or premenstrual syndrome; improved endometrial bleeding patterns; or amenorrhea. The protective effect of the combined pill against ovarian and endometrial cancer is perceived as an advantage by providers and enhances continuation rates among well-informed women. Contraceptive methods that reduce the risk of breast cancer and prostate cancer would be enormously attractive to large numbers of women and men, respectively. Likewise, a contraceptive method that also confers protection against HIV infection and other STIs is likely to have widespread benefit. The challenge of developing products that have multiple effects (contraceptive and noncontraceptive) is substantial, but this goal is worthy of pursuit given the potential value of such an agent. Clinical evaluation and registration of a single product for two indications are more complex and time-consuming, but they have been accomplished for some therapeutic agents. Furthermore, several formulations that exhibit both spermicidal and microbicidal effects are now in clinical trials.

Recommendation 9: During the development of drugs and drug delivery systems, efforts should be made to discover, enhance, and promote the noncontraceptive health benefits of existing and new methods of contraception. Intensified efforts to develop contraceptive methods that are prophylactic for HIV infection and other STIs are especially needed.

STRATEGIES FOR RESEARCH SUCCESS

Expand Public–Private Partnerships

Public–private partnerships, such as the International AIDS Vaccine Initiative and the Global Alliance for Tuberculosis Drug Development, have significant track records in attracting and retaining industry interest in a particular scientific area. These partnerships target disease areas that large multinational corporations are reluctant to consider because of unsolved access problems, negative public relations, unresolved intellectual property rights issues, and difficult scientific hurdles.

This was the rationale for the initiation of several productive partnerships established since the release of the 1996 IOM report, including the Consortium for Industrial Collaboration in Contraceptive Research (CICCR) and the Global Microbicide Project (GMP). External review committees gave high marks to CICCR and GMP and to their individual program areas for progress toward their stated objectives. Thus, these programs, which were initiated to support innovative high-risk research, to identify novel targets, or to focus new efforts in neglected areas, could serve as models for public–private collaborations in contraceptive development.

The committee concludes that the creation of public–private partnerships is an important mechanism to advance research in reproductive health and contraception. The complementary scientific strengths and focus of the not-for-profit and for-profit sectors are necessary to ensure rapid progress in the translation of lead compounds to products. The support of philanthropic foundations in promoting this concept is commendable, and further collaboration between public and private organizations active in the field would be worthwhile.

Recommendation 10: Expand public–private partnerships that draw on the complementary strengths of the public-sector agencies, industry, foundations, consumer groups, and other organizations to expedite the translation of lead compounds into contraceptive products.

Increase the Participation of Developing Countries

Nongovernmental organizations, governmental public health agencies, universities, research institutions, medical research councils, and industry in developing countries can make valuable contributions to contraceptive development in several ways. First, institutions in developing countries can clearly play a role in assessing contraceptive acceptability among users in these countries, for example by determining the preferred routes of administration and delivery vehicles or systems. Second, some developing countries have active research programs that have already made contributions to contraception, including work on injectables in Brazil and male contraceptives in China. Third, a number of developing countries have flourishing pharmaceutical industries, some of which already meet Good Manufacturing Practice standards. Locally produced products may also be more widely accepted in some countries. Fourth, many institutions in developing countries are involved in clinical trials of contraceptives. The cost of clinical trials is generally lower in these countries, and enrollment targets are often achieved faster. This valuable resource could be expanded if funding were available not only for strengthening capacity but also for ensuring that clinical trial sites meet Good Clinical Practice standards.

Establishment of collaborations between developed and developing countries has been supported by the World Health Organization Department of Reproductive Health and Research and its network of collaborating centers, the Indo-U.S. Joint Working Group on Contraceptives and Reproductive Health Research, the Andrew W. Mellon Foundation's "twinning program" for collaboration between centers of excellence in the United States and developing countries (which will soon cease), and the Fogarty International Center competitive research grants for foreign investigators who are collaborating with a U.S. investigator. The Global Health in Research Initiative provides competitive reentry grants to foreign scholars who have had postdoctoral training in the United States sponsored by Fogarty International Center training grants. Programs such as CONRAD, the Consortium for Industrial Collaboration in Contraceptive Research, the GMP, Family Health International, the Program for Appropriate Technology in Health, the Population Council, and the World Health Organization also have active collaborations with institutions worldwide, not just for clinical trials but also for preclinical activities and feasibility and proof-of-concept studies.

Recommendation 11: Facilitate collaboration between organizations in developed and developing countries in contraceptive development, clinical testing, and understanding of acceptability of methods. Specifically:

- Use centers of excellence worldwide, especially in developing countries, to incorporate knowledge of local needs and preferences into research on methods that will be acceptable to different cultures.
- Collaborate with pharmaceutical companies in developing countries to facilitate the rapid development of new contraceptive agents.
- Involve sites in developing countries with expertise in conducting basic and clinical research on new contraceptives, and where

necessary, assist these sites in meeting Good Clinical Practice standards.

Increase Clinical and Scientific Training and Career Development in Contraception

A cadre of scientists and physicians dedicated to contraceptive development is needed to implement the contraceptive research agenda. Although quantitative data on investigator training or the workforce in the specific field of contraception were not readily available, the committee believes that there is a paucity of such individuals in academe, that the average age of those who are active is rising, and that prospects for new entrants into the field are currently bleak. A major challenge is to identify, attract, train, and support the career development of young investigators in basic, translational, clinical, and social sciences as well as project management who have an interest in and appreciation for the multidisciplinary issues surrounding fertility regulation. More postdoctoral training opportunities are needed, and trainees who complete a rigorous program should be recognized as experts through learned societies or organizations. To encourage young investigators, there must also be the promise of adequate opportunities to obtain research funding. Given the long period of time required in this field to make substantive contributions that may lead to new products, junior or midlevel faculty need the promise of adequate support. The academic community itself must also appreciate the unique features of contraceptive development research so as not to penalize those who pursue activities that may be viewed as being outside the traditional path (e.g., applied research or team-based research).

Recommendation 12: Establish, support, and recognize new programs for training and career advancement in contraceptive research and clinical practice.

- Establish new basic and clinical fellowship programs for postdoctoral training in contraception.
- Establish endowed professorships with long-term funding for contraceptive research.

Establish Resources and Mechanisms to Strategically Manage and Coordinate Efforts

Women and men at different stages of life and from different populations have different notions of the appropriate forms of contraception as well as variable access to health care. The difficulty of identifying promising targets for multiple populations is compounded by the multiplicity of disciplines involved in contraceptive development, the high cost of product development, and the complexity of product introduction and monitoring. Decisions about which targets to pursue and which to abandon would be facilitated by access to the combined wisdom of multiple disciplines and parties with diverse interests. At present, there is no central coordinating body, information source, or interagency working group on the specific topic of contraception. Collaboration occurs only on an ad hoc basis through the major governmental, nongovernmental, and not-for-profit participants in contraceptive research and development.

In contrast, a model exists in the related field of microbicide development. The Alliance for Microbicide Development acts as a clearinghouse for all new information on microbicides and keeps an up-to-date database showing the progress of all current lead compounds through the research and development pipeline. One level of the database is open to all and contains only information that is in the public domain or that is not proprietary. The second level contains proprietary information about the various lead compounds and is open only to developers and their collaborators and to potential funders.

Another strategy for improving communication among the many parties with an interest in this rapidly changing scientific field is a roundtable or forum. While an Alliance for Contraceptive Development would collect resource material and disseminate information, a Forum on Contraceptive Research would provide a mechanism to facilitate integration of the activities of different stakeholders. This approach has been used successfully in other areas of biomedical research, such as microbial threats and clinical research. A forum on contraceptive research and development would provide a mechanism by which interested parties from the academic, industrial, consumer, philanthropic, health, and federal research and regulatory perspectives could be convened to discuss sensitive and difficult issues of mutual interest in a neutral setting. The purpose would be to foster dialogue and discussion across sectors and institutions and to illuminate issues but not necessarily resolve them. The forum could also identify and suggest topics for separate, independent study by other groups. Specific agenda topics would be determined by the forum membership and would incorporate the interests of all parties and focus on issues of broad concern.

Recommendation 13: Create organizations to promote communication among the many parties interested in contraceptive research and to serve as a clearinghouse for information on contraceptive research.

• Establish an ongoing Forum on Contraceptive Research and Development at which the different sectors and institutions involved in contraceptive research can discuss topics of common interest.

- Create an Alliance for Contraceptive Development, modeled after the Alliance for Microbicide Development, to serve as an information-gathering and information exchange mechanism in the contraceptive research field. The Alliance should:
  — Create and operate a listserve or other mechanism by which scientists involved in basic research on reproductive biology and contraceptive research and development can communicate (e.g., by providing an opportunity to pose questions or problems requiring generation of laboratory data on compounds, which other listserv members might answer).
  — Use the power of the Internet to provide resource information to scientists regarding drug delivery efforts in other research areas, analysis of current delivery systems in the contraceptive field, and contact information for contract laboratories.
  — Stimulate and maintain public awareness and support for contraceptive research and development by providing ongoing information through an Internet site reporting the progress of research activities.

CONCLUSION

The development of new contraceptives benefits men, women, and families worldwide, because contraception is one of the most effective means of improving reproductive health and quality of life. Governments and institutions worldwide can and do make valuable contributions to efforts aimed at developing and disseminating contraceptive technologies, but support from the United States, the largest single funder of biomedical research, is important for meaningful progress in the field. Responding to both national and international unmet needs with respect to contraception is a matter of self-interest for the United States, and deploying the nation's intellectual and technical resources to address the problem of fertility control and family planning worldwide helps fulfill the humanitarian responsibility of the United States. Success in this area can provide indirect benefits to all countries of the world, including the United States, through improvements in political and economic order and through better stewardship of the environment, leading to improved quality of life globally.

The extraordinary recent advances in science and technology provide unprecedented opportunities to develop completely new approaches to contraception. Progress in the field will depend on adequate and sustained funding, as well as a new influx of broadly trained scientists and clinicians focused on contraceptive research; failure to immediately capitalize on these opportunities through new research initiatives would be tragic for the future generations of the world. Now is the time to address the critical needs and issues identified in this report and to ensure that future investments in contraceptive research, discovery, and development are brought to fruition to improve the lives and health of people worldwide.

REFERENCES

Global Health Council. 2002. *Promises to Keep: The Toll of Unintended Pregnancies on Women's Lives in the Developing World.* Washington, DC: Global Health Council.
Institute of Medicine. 1996. *Contraceptive Research and Development: Looking to the Future.* Harrison PF, Rosenfield A, eds. Washington, DC: National Academy Press.

1

Introduction

Family planning is a socially beneficial activity that affects the well-being of women, men, children, families, and society as a whole. The benefits of planned fertility include the more effective intergenerational transfer of resources, resulting in improved child health and development (Lee, 2003); increased longevity and empowerment of women, with the attendant economic benefits to the family and the community; and a reduced lifetime risk of chronic illness or death from a pregnancy-related condition. Contraception, when practiced with barrier methods, also lessens the likelihood of sexually transmitted diseases. By consciously practicing family planning, couples can choose to contribute to the overall health, stability, and economy of their families and their communities.

Conversely, the consequences of unintended pregnancy are quite serious, imposing significant burdens on children, women, men, and families (reviewed by the Institute of Medicine, 1995). The child born from an unplanned conception is at greater risk of low birth weight, dying in its first year of life, being abused, and not receiving sufficient resources for healthy development. An unplanned conception also exposes women to the usual health risks of pregnancy, which can include maternal death. Closely spaced births pose additional risks for the mother and child. In a study that controlled for socioeconomic and demographic differences, it was found that women who spaced childbearing at 27- to 32-month intervals were 2.5 times more likely to survive childbirth than women who gave birth at 9- to 14-month intervals. Children born 3 to 4 years after a previous birth were found to be 2.3 times more likely to survive the first year of life than children born less than 2 years after a previous birth

(Rinehart et al., 2002). When a pregnancy is unplanned, the mother also has a greater risk of depression and of being physically abused, and her relationship with her partner is at greater risk of dissolution. Both the mother and the father of the child may suffer economic hardship and may fail to achieve their educational and career goals. Given these issues, a woman experiencing an unintended pregnancy may also face the decision to have an abortion.

Unintended pregnancy is frequent and widespread in the United States (Institute of Medicine, 1995) and the world (Global Health Council, 2002). In the United States, about half of all pregnancies are unintended at the time of conception (Henshaw, 1998; Institute of Medicine, 1995). According to a recent analysis by the Global Health Council, the world's 1.3 billion women between the ages of 15 and 45 experienced more than 1.2 billion pregnancies in the 6 years between 1995 and 2000.[1] Of these, more than 300 million—or more than one-quarter—were unintended. Unintended pregnancy affects all segments of society—it is not just a problem of teenagers or unmarried women, poor women or minorities, or women living in the developing world. For example, a survey of more than 14,000 French households revealed that 33 percent of pregnancies occurring over a 5-year period were unplanned, half of which were terminated by abortion. Sixty-five percent of the unplanned pregnancies occurred among women using contraception (Bajos et al., 2003). A survey in the United States found that 50 percent of unintended pregnancies occurred among couples using some form of contraception (Henshaw, 1998).

Poor women in developing countries bear the greatest burden with regard to maternal mortality and morbidity due to unplanned pregnancies. The lifetime risk of dying during pregnancy and childbirth in these countries is several hundred times higher than that in wealthier nations (1 in 4,000 in North America and Europe versus 1 in 15 in Africa). Maternal mortality is highest in countries where women are least likely to have access to modern contraceptive services (Global Health Council, 2002). In Burkina Faso, where only 4 percent of women use family planning methods, 1 in 14 will die of maternal causes over the course of her

---

[1]The Global Health Council compiled a country-by-country profile of all 227 countries in the world, based on the best available statistics from the U.S. Census Bureau, United Nations agencies, country reports, and specialized surveys carried out by a variety of respected research organizations. For each country and each year, data were generated on the number of pregnancies that occurred, the number that ended in miscarriages and abortions, and the number carried to term. For each of these, the data sources were used to assess the number that resulted from unintended pregnancies and the number of unintended pregnancies that resulted in the death of the mother.

lifetime. In Brazil, the opposite is true; nearly three-quarters of the female population regularly use family planning services, and their lifetime risk of maternal mortality is considerably lower: 1 in 130 (Global Health Council, 2002). In Russia, abortion has long been the traditional method of family planning (Gadasina, 1997), and Russia has the highest abortion rate in the world.[2] Although pregnancy terminations are freely available, contraception is not. Nonetheless, even with the easy availability of abortion services, an estimated 15 percent of procedures are performed in illegal private facilities. The lack of contraceptive choices has resulted in excess maternal mortality—nearly one-third of maternal deaths in Russia are estimated to be due to abortion procedures—and an explosion in sexually transmitted infections (Karelova, 1999; Parfitt, 2003).

Although the number of live births has stabilized at about 131 million per year worldwide, the number of women dying each year as a result of unintended pregnancy has increased since 1995. Over the 6 years examined, nearly 700,000 women died as a result of unintended pregnancies. Although more than one-third died from problems associated with pregnancy, labor, and delivery, the majority—more than 400,000—died as a result of complications resulting from abortions carried out under unsafe and often illegal conditions. An unintended pregnancy often leads to the decision to have an abortion. Furthermore, for every maternal death, an estimated 30 additional women suffer pregnancy-related health problems that are frequently permanently debilitating (Global Health Council, 2002).

The death of a mother is emotionally, socially, and economically destructive to families and communities (Global Health Council, 2002). In developing nations, where an estimated 98 percent of pregnancy-related deaths take place, the loss of a mother translates into the increased likelihood that surviving family members will not be able to properly care for existing children, and such children have a much greater risk of dying themselves (Steiner et al., 2000). Moreover, because these women typically die between the ages of 15 and 45, elevated rates of maternal mortality represent a significant threat to the broader socioeconomic systems (reviewed by the Global Health Council, 2002).

CONTRACEPTIVE USE

Contraceptive use in developing countries has increased greatly since the 1960s and in many cases is now approaching the levels observed in

---

[2]See The Library of Congress—Country Studies, 1996, available online at http://www.1upinfo.com/country-guide-study/russia/russia65.html (accessed October 2003).

developed countries (overall rates of use, 60 and 70 percent of couples, respectively). Worldwide, more than 580 million women use modern methods of contraception (Figure 1.1), contributing to a large drop in the total fertility rate in developing countries (United Nations Development Programme, 2003; United Nations Population Fund, 2001; World Bank, 2003; World Health Organization, 2003). The trend is notable not only for its demographic impact but also for its ability to free women to pursue a productive life in addition to a reproductive life. However, studies show that more than 120 million people around the world do not use any form of contraception, even though they report that they are sexually active and do not wish to become pregnant (Figure 1.1).

Although a number of effective reversible and nonreversible contraceptive methods exist (barrier methods, hormonal methods, intrauterine devices, and contraceptive sterilization), all have shortcomings in the form of failure rates and undesirable side effects that lead to the discontinuation of reversible methods. WHO's recent warning[3] against the use of spermicides by women at high risk of HIV infection may lead to further reduction in the use of barrier methods. The effectiveness of many contraceptives depends on correct and consistent use, which can be difficult for people to achieve (Trussell and Stewart, 1998). Indeed, U.S. women and their partners relying on reversible means of contraception and those using no contraception contribute roughly equally to the pool of unintended pregnancies. In the United States, the 7 percent of women who are at risk for unintended pregnancy and who use no method of contraception account for about half of all unintended pregnancies that occur each year (Henshaw, 1998). The remaining 50 percent of all unintended pregnancies occurred among 93 percent of at-risk U.S. couples practicing some form of contraception, partly reflecting the inconsistent use of effective methods. The same pattern is true in other developed countries (Bajos et al., 2003; Darroch et al., 2001).

In addition, most currently available methods have discontinuation rates approaching 50 percent after 1 year of use, usually because of side effects (Rosenberg et al., 1995; Trussell and Vaughan, 1999). When women discontinue highly effective methods, they usually choose a less effective method. For example, one study showed that 70 percent of women who discontinue oral contraceptives begin using a less effective method, and 20 percent use no contraceptive method at all (Rosenberg et al., 1995). Moreover, women who continue using a method often do so despite the

---

[3]See http://www.who.int/reproductive-health/family_planning/updates.html (accessed November 2003).

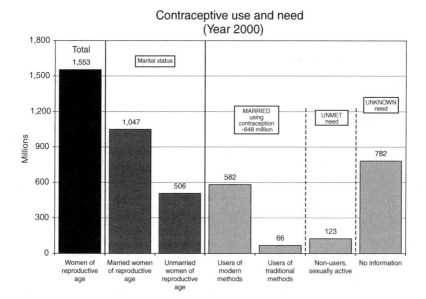

FIGURE 1.1 Contraceptive use and need worldwide. Traditional methods include withdrawal, periodic abstinence, and other non-supply-related methods. Modern methods include hormonal contraceptives and barrier methods such as diaphragms, condoms, and intrauterine devices.

Column 1: Total number of women of reproductive age (15-49) is 1.553 billion in the year 2000 (Population Division of the Department of Economic and Social Affairs of the United Nations Secretariat, 2003).

Column 2: Total number of women of reproductive age (15-49) married or in union is 1.047 billion (Population Division of the Department of Economic and Social Affairs of the United Nations Secretariat, 2002).

Column 3: Unmarried women of reproductive age number 506 million (subtracting Column 2 from Column 1). This figure is included because we know very little about the needs of these women and if or how they are being met. Some of them are sexually active and using contraceptive methods, some are sexually active and are not using any method of family planning, some may wish to conceive, and some are not sexually active.

Columns 4 and 5: Married women using contraceptive methods, separated according to "modern" and "traditional" (Population Division of the Department of Economic and Social Affairs of the United Nations Secretariat, 2002).

Column 6: 123 million: Unmet need as defined by the number of women wishing to space or limit births but not currently using a method of contraception. This number includes married and unmarried women in developing countries (excluding China) and the former Soviet Union, but not the West and so is probably an underestimation. Numbers in other columns are world-wide (Ross and Winfrey International Family Planning perspectives, 2002).

Column 7: Use and needs for 782 million women are unaccounted for in the graph (subtract Columns 4, 5, and 6 from Column 1). Their needs may be met, unmet, or unknown, depending on their sexual activity and desire for pregnancy.

presence of unwanted side effects, which they tolerate in return for pregnancy prevention. Thus, continuation rates are not a surrogate for acceptability (Severy, 1999; Severy and Thapa, 1994). The cultural, personal, or political unacceptability of the various methods also can contribute to a lack of contraceptive use.

Access to effective methods may also be quite limited for many segments of society, especially those in developing countries with inadequate resources for health care. Beginning in 1998, 20 U.S. states have required that health insurers cover all contraceptives approved by the FDA (Alan Guttmacher Institute, 2003). However, at the federal level, legislation introduced in 1997, 1999, and 2001 to mandate such coverage was never brought to a vote. Further, an estimated 43.6 million people lacked health insurance for all of 2002 (U.S. Department of Commerce, 2003) and none of these people would have benefited from a mandated coverage of contraception by health insurers.

Even if total contraceptive prevalence were to remain the same, the need for access to effective contraceptive methods will continue to rise as increasing numbers of people worldwide attain reproductive age. Worldwide, about 60 percent of couples at risk for pregnancy use contraceptives, but in some developing countries, the rates of contraceptive use are much lower. Countries in sub-Saharan Africa, for example, have contraceptive use rates of only about 20 percent.[4] Although the population growth rate is slowing and in fact has become negative in a number of Western countries, the population of the world as a whole continues to rise, particularly in developing countries. As a result, during the next decade, 600 million girls will become adolescents, which will be the largest cohort of young women in human history (Global Health Council, 2002). Because these young women will be from diverse backgrounds, there will be an urgent need for a larger variety of contraceptive methods. Moreover, it is now well appreciated that there is no "perfect" contraceptive because the contraception needs of women and men change over the reproductive and family life cycles. Methods are needed for child spacing as well as permanent pregnancy prevention, for adolescents as well as those approaching menopause, for postpartum and breast-feeding women, for women and men with medical conditions that restrict the contraceptive that they can use, for men and women with few resources, and for men and women whose personal situations make correct and consistent use difficult. In addition, the development of new dual protection methods—those that protect against pregnancy as well as against HIV/AIDS and other sexually transmitted infections—would be highly benefi-

---

[4]According to 2002 data of the United Nations Population Division.

cial, since the HIV/AIDS pandemic threatens world health and continues to devastate sub-Saharan Africa and Asia. Clearly, there is an enormous unmet need for effective and acceptable family planning worldwide. For many men, women, children, families, and communities, the negative consequences of not meeting family planning needs are high.

Cost, accessibility, and consistent and correct use of existing methods still present enormous challenges to international family planning efforts in particular. Although there is value in improving the characteristics and means of delivery of current methods, there is also urgency in proceeding with new research on and the development of new methods to meet the range of contraceptive needs throughout the world and across the human life span. The usual time line from basic research through target identification and then to product introduction of 10 to 14 years means that an effort initiated today would barely be on track to meet the aforementioned contraception needs of the coming decade. The development of new contraceptives that increase the range of options available to women and men worldwide would improve the lives of families everywhere.

In 1996, the Institute of Medicine (1996) issued its most recent of several reports assessing the state of contraceptive research and development. That report exposed and analyzed the reasons for the apparent lack of activity and progress in the field since the first "contraceptive revolution," which began in the 1950s and 1960s, when most of the current contraceptive methods were initially developed (Institute of Medicine, 1996). Many of the recommendations put forth in that report are as relevant today as they were in 1996, but the recent unprecedented advances in science and technology warrant a fresh examination of the research goals and agenda in field of contraception. Although progress has been made in the intervening years, contraceptive modalities recently developed or introduced are mainly variations on preexisting approaches. Furthermore, progress in some areas thought to be promising in 1996 (e.g., immunocontraception) has been minimal, whereas new discoveries point to promising new opportunities. Moreover, there is still a great need to reenergize the field and to translate significant observations from the science of reproductive biology to practical application in fertility regulation. Many barriers remain, but the progress that has been made is evidence that they can be surmounted with committed resources and hard work.

COMMITTEE CHARGE

The current IOM committee was charged with recommending priority areas for future research and development in the field of contraception. To accomplish that goal, the committee assumed three main tasks in this study:

- In basic science, to identify opportunities derived from recent advances in biomedical research.
- In the product development process, to propose new strategies and frameworks for contraceptive development.
- In implementation, to describe the resources, infrastructure, and coordination needed to achieve success.

With respect to science, revolutionary changes have occurred in basic biomedical research, materials sciences, and drug delivery since publication of the 1996 IOM report. The advances in biomedical research have provided exciting new opportunities for studying the basic biology of reproduction, which could in turn lead to the discovery of new targets for contraception. In particular, the tools and technologies of genomics, proteomics, lipidomics, and glycomics have great potential for identifying targets that could facilitate the development of radically new approaches to contraception. Novel approaches for the development and delivery of drugs and other products could also provide new insights into ways to create innovative contraceptives once potential targets have been identified. Despite these advances, however, there has been flagging interest in contraceptive development—not only in the pharmaceutical industry but also in the broader scientific community—that must be revived if these innovations are to generate products that satisfy the demand for safe, effective, and convenient contraceptives.

Regarding the product development process, many obstacles to contraceptive development were identified in past IOM reports, particularly the 1996 report, and many continue to plague the field. However, new paradigms for science, including large-scale science, have emerged in the past few years, along with new models for public–private collaboration.

In terms of implementation, new parties are interested in the process of contraceptive development and dissemination, and new global consortia are also dealing with reproductive health. These new participants offer unique opportunities to move contraceptive development forward if there is an expansion of the number and the breadth of expertise of scientists and clinicians dedicated to contraceptive research and development. Those who are active in the field are nearing retirement, with prospects for new blood seemingly bleak without a widespread commitment to and enthusiasm about contraceptive research and development. A major challenge is to identify, attract, train, and support the career development of individuals who have an appreciation for the multidisciplinary issues surrounding fertility regulation. This will require a significant departure from the current ways in which investigators are trained as well as a specialized environment for carrying out research in this area. These topics will be addressed in greater detail in the remaining chapters of this report.

FRAMEWORK OF THE REPORT

Chapter 2 provides an overview of technological advances that have revolutionized the fields of biomedical research, drug discovery, and drug development and that could thus have a tremendous impact on contraceptive research and development. The committee examines ways in which the new methods can be used to identify and validate targets before drug development.

Chapter 3 describes the challenges associated with product identification and development, once potential new targets for contraceptive development have been identified, and suggests a variety of approaches to stimulate and speed progress in translational research and drug development.

Chapter 4 examines the role of the social and behavioral sciences in shaping the pursuit of leads that are likely to find a receptive set of users and that are appropriate to particular populations or circumstances. This chapter also examines ways to improve the use and acceptability of current and new contraceptives, such as enhancing and promoting other health benefits beyond pregnancy prevention.

Chapter 5 delineates a variety of strategies that can be used to capitalize on advances in science and technology and to overcome remaining obstacles to progress in contraceptive research and development.

Because of the important role of the 1996 IOM report *Contraceptive Research and Development: Looking to the Future* as a foundation for the committee's work, an update on developments that have occurred since that report was published is included in Appendix A. The agenda for and participants in the committee's workshop are provided in Appendix B, and a short biography of each member of the committee is presented in Appendix C.

REFERENCES

Alan Guttmacher Institute. 2003. *State Policies in Brief: Insurance Coverage of Contraceptives.* [Online]. Available: http://www.agi-usa.org/pubs/spib_ICC.pdf [accessed November 2003].

Bajos N, Leridon H, Goulard H, Oustry P, Job-Spira N. 2003. Contraception: from accessibility to efficiency. *Hum Reprod* 18(5):994–999.

Darroch JE, Singh S, Frost JJ. 2001. Differences in teenage pregnancy rates among five developed countries: the roles of sexual activity and contraceptive use. *Fam Plann Perspect* 33(6):244–250, 281.

Gadasina A. 1997. Struggling to survive in Russia. *Plan Parent Chall* (1-2):40–42.

Global Health Council. 2002. *Promises to Keep: The Toll of Unintended Pregnancies on Women's Lives in the Developing World.* Washington, DC: Global Health Council.

Henshaw SK. 1998. Unintended pregnancy in the United States. *Fam Plann Perspect* 30(1):24–29, 46.

Institute of Medicine. 1995. *The Best Intentions: Unintended Pregnancy and the Well-Being of Children and Families*. Brown S, Eisenberg L, eds. Washington, DC: National Academy Press.

Institute of Medicine. 1996. *Contraceptive Research and Development: Looking to the Future*. Harrison PF, Rosenfield A, eds. Washington, DC: National Academy Press.

Karelova GN. 1999. A reduction of abortions. Russian Federation. The Hague Forum. *Integration* (60):29.

Lee RD. 2003. Rethinking the evolutionary theory of aging: transfers, not births, shape senescence in social species. *Proc Natl Acad Sci U S A* 100(16):9637–9642.

Parfitt T. 2003. Russia moves to curb abortion rates. *Lancet* 362(9388):968.

Population Division of the Department of Economic and Social Affairs of the United Nations Secretariat. 2002. *World Contraceptive Use, 2001*. New York: United Nations.

Population Division of the Department of Economic and Social Affairs of the United Nations Secretariat. 2003. *World Population Prospects: The 2002 Revision*. New York: United Nations. [Online]. Available: http://www.unpopulation.org/ [accessed December 2003].

Rinehart W, Compton AW, Rigby HM. 2002. Three to Five Saves Lives. *Population Reports* 30(3):1.

Rosenberg MJ, Waugh MS, Meehan TE. 1995. Use and misuse of oral contraceptives: risk indicators for poor pill taking and discontinuation. *Contraception* 51(5):283–288.

Ross JA, Winfrey WL. 2002. Unmet need for contraception in the developing world and the former Soviet Union: an updated estimate. *International Family Planning Perspectives* 28(3):138–143.

Severy LJ. 1999. Acceptability as a critical component of clinical trials. *Adv Pop* 3:103–122.

Severy LJ, Thapa S. 1994. Preferences and tolerance as determinants of contraceptive acceptability. *Adv Pop* 2:119–139.

Steiner MJ, Taylor DJ, Feldblum PJ, Wheeless AJ. 2000. How well do male latex condoms work? Pregnancy outcome during one menstrual cycle of use. *Contraception* 62(6):315–319.

Trussell J, Stewart F. 1998. Contraceptive efficacy. In: Hatcher RA, Trussell J, Stewart F, Cates W, Stewart GK, Guest F, Kowal D. *Contraceptive Technology*. 17th rev. ed. New York: Ardent Media.

Trussell J, Vaughan B. 1999. Contraceptive failure, method-related discontinuation and resumption of use: results from the 1995 National Survey of Family Growth. *Fam Plann Perspect* 31(2):64–72, 93.

United Nations Development Programme. 2003. *Human Development Report 2003: Millennium Development Goals: A Compact among Nations to End Human Poverty*. [Online]. Available: http://hdr.undp.org/reports/view_reports.cfm?year=2003 [accessed August 2003].

United Nations Population Fund. 2001. *Annual Report 2001*. [Online]. Available: http://www.unfpa.org/about/report/2001/index.htm [accessed August 2003].

U.S. Department of Commerce, U.S. Census Bureau. 2003. *Health Insurance Coverage in the United States 2002*. [Online]. Available: http://www.census.gov/prod/2003pubs/p60-223.pdf [accessed November 2003].

World Bank. 2003. *World Development Report 2003: Sustainable Development in a Dynamic World*. [Online]. Available: http://econ.worldbank.org/wdr/wdr2003/ [accessed August 2003].

World Health Organization. 2003. *The World Health Report 2002*. [Online]. Available: http://www.who.int/whr/en/ [accessed August 2003].

2

Target Discovery and Validation

Major advances in biomedical research have occurred in the last decade of the 20th century, and these advances will be reflected in improvements in human health care as the 21st century proceeds. Technological advances in the area of genomics have permitted the complete or nearly complete sequencing of the genomes of several species, including humans as well as model organisms, such as the fruit fly, nematode worm, pufferfish, rat, and mouse. Advances in computational abilities and bioinformatics, along with the development of large-scale, high-throughput technologies such as DNA microarrays, have helped to define tissue- and cell-specific patterns of gene transcription, referred to as "transcriptomes." New tools for sequencing proteins have also provided information on the complete protein complements of cellular components, referred to as "proteomics."

In parallel with these contributions, studies in "functional genomics" that use a variety of technologies in vitro and in vivo have helped to identify and characterize essential and novel functions of genes. In the process of performing these various analyses, thousands of genes have been found to be expressed in the cells and tissues that function in reproduction. At least several hundred of these genes appear to be unique to reproductive cells and tissues, and more than 200 human genes or their counterparts in model organisms have been shown to play roles in reproduction in vivo (Matzuk and Lamb, 2002). Because genes that are highly or exclusively expressed in the reproductive tract continue to be discovered, it is likely that additional functional genomics studies will validate these gene products as putative contraceptive targets in men and women.

Mutations in a particular gene or genes that lead to an infertility phenotype in model organisms would suggest that specific modulation of the same gene product in humans could also, theoretically, result in a contraceptive effect. The more specific the expression and, more importantly, the more specific the function of these genes in the reproductive tract, the less likely it is that a new reproductive tract-specific contraceptive would have unwanted side effects. Furthermore, genes whose protein products function as receptors, enzymes, and ion channels or transporter proteins, classes of molecules that have been targeted most commonly by pharmaceuticals (Figure 2.1), would likely be of greatest interest for developing new contraceptive drugs.

This chapter provides a brief overview of several of the new methodologies used in basic biomedical research that could be brought to bear on the identification and validation of novel targets for contraception. Other methods or technologies might also make valuable contributions to the discovery and validation of new targets, but it was not possible to provide a comprehensive review of all possible scientific approaches to contraceptive research here. The chapter focuses primarily on early stage discovery approaches to research in reproductive biology, which should be viewed

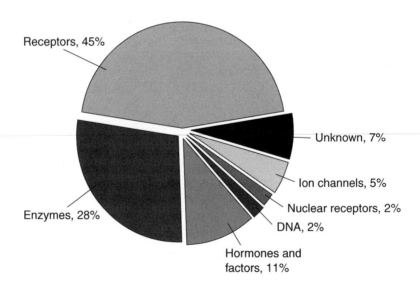

FIGURE 2.1 Molecular targets of drug therapy, with classification according to biochemical criteria. Based on modern standard work in pharmacology, the molecular targets of all known drugs that have been characterized as safe and effective have been collected and listed according to their biochemical nature. SOURCE: Drews, 2000.

as a long-term investment in the field, as it will likely take many years, perhaps even decades, to translate the new knowledge into clinically useful and acceptable contraceptives. The chapter also includes a few examples of promising targets that have already been identified and that could potentially be used to develop new contraceptives in a somewhat shorter time frame. Again, a comprehensive list of possible targets was not possible, but a general overview of potential contraceptive targets is provided in the following section.

OVERVIEW OF REPRODUCTIVE BIOLOGY

Reproduction is a complex process involving many different specialized cells, tissues, and organs in both the male and the female (Institute of Medicine, 1996; reviewed in Matzuk and Lamb, 2002). Figure 2.2 provides an overview of the male and female reproductive processes that could potentially be targeted by contraceptives. Recent advances in basic biological research have provided a better understanding of these processes than ever before, and examples of the many genes that may play an important role in reproduction at various stages are shown in Figures 2.3 and 2.4.

A small number of germ cells are set aside from somatic cells early in embryogenesis, where they usually remain in an undifferentiated quiescent state while somatic cells are dividing and forming tissues and organs. In order to form gametes, they must then begin to proliferate and enter meiosis, a process that is unique to germ cells and is required to halve the number of chromosomes in a gamete's nucleus so that it can combine with another haploid gamete at fertilization.

Male spermatogenesis is initiated postnatally and is a continuous process characterized by three specific functional phases: proliferation, meiosis, and spermiogenesis. Proliferating cells known as spermatogonia undergo differentiation and enter meiosis as spermatocytes. Once male germ cells complete meiosis to achieve a haploid chromosomal complement, they are called spermatids. Spermatids undergo a process of cellular differentiation known as spermiogenesis, progressing from round to elongated spermatids, and culminating in the development of spermatozoa. After spermatogenesis, spermatozoa are released from the Sertoli cells into the seminiferous tubule lumen.

In the female, gametes develop in structures called follicles within the ovary. Oogenesis begins as follicles form during prenatal life in humans, and arrests at an early stage of meiosis. Recruitment of individual follicles leads to further growth and development of oocytes, with a resumption of meiosis, and culminates in ovulation, or release of the oocyte into the oviduct. At that point, the oocyte arrests again in a late stage of meiosis

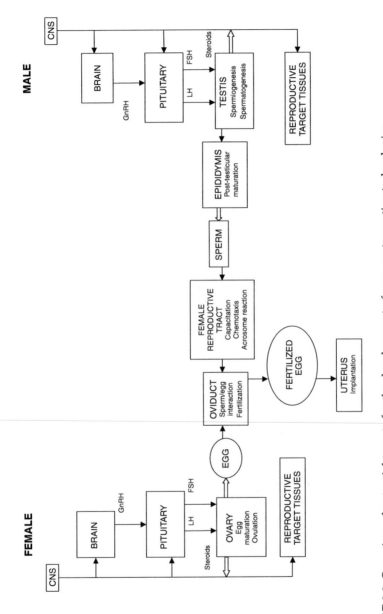

FIGURE 2.2 Overview of potential targets for the development of new contraceptive technologies.
NOTE: CNS = central nervous system, GnRH = gonadotropin releasing hormone, LH = luteinizing hormone, FSH = follicle stimulating hormone.
SOURCE: Adapted from Institute of Medicine, 1996.

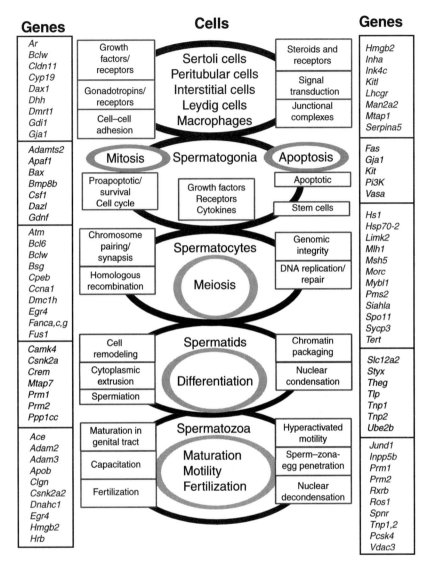

FIGURE 2.3 Genes involved in the regulation of male reproduction in the mouse. Spermatogenesis requires a complex interaction of the various cellular compartments of the testis (seminiferous epithelium containing spermatogenic cells, Sertoli cells, and peritubular myoid cells; the interstitial cell compartment containing the steroidogenic Leydig cells, macrophages, and other interstitial cells; and the vasculature). Targeted mutation of the genes shown affects specific testicular cell types and reproductive function, resulting in male infertility or subfertility in the mouse.
SOURCE: Matzuk and Lamb, 2002.

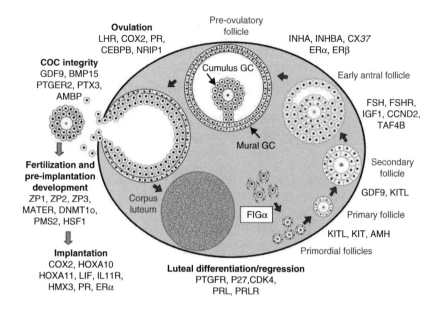

FIGURE 2.4 Female fertility proteins. Knockout mouse models have defined key proteins that function at various stages of follicle formation, folliculogenesis, ovulation, and post-ovulatory events. Several proteins are needed for primordial follicle formation, oocyte and granulose cell (GC) growth and differentiation, ovulation, and the integrity of the cumulus oocyte complex (COC). SOURCE: Matzuk and Lamb, 2002.

until fertilized by a sperm. In contrast to males, the formation of follicles in females results in a finite endowment of oocytes. Over the course of a woman's lifetime, there is a precipitous decline in the number of oocytes. The roughly 7 million germ cells in a 20-week-old fetus are reduced to 2 million oocytes at birth, and eventually to 300,000 oocytes at puberty. Only about 400 of those will ever undergo ovulation.

Despite this sexual difference in meiosis, many regulators of the process are common to the germ cells of both males and females. Both are controlled from the brain through the production of gonadotropin-releasing hormone (GnRH) by the hypothalamus. GnRH in turn stimulates the anterior pituitary to secrete luteinizing hormone (LH) and follicle-stimulating hormone (FSH), both of which are required for normal gamete development as well as steroid hormone production (such as testosterone, estrogen, and progesterone). Chemical communication between developing gametes and their supportive somatic cells via growth factors and cytokines is also essential for egg and sperm production.

When sperm leave the testis, they must undergo more morphologic and biochemical changes before they are capable of fertilization. These final developments take place in the epididymis, which also serves as a sperm storage reservoir. During maturation, much of the sperm surface appears to be remodeled. Products secreted by the epithelium of the epididymis mediate these changes. Although the precise components of this epididymal fluid have not been fully identified, it is known that its complex composition changes dramatically along the length of the epididymal tubule.

The sperm maturation process continues when sperm enter the female reproductive tract. It is here that they undergo a process known as capacitation, during which they acquire the ability to fertilize an egg. For fertilization to take place, sperm must be motile and make their way to the oviduct, a step that may involve chemical signals from the egg or components of the female reproductive tract (Inaba, 2003). Once a sperm comes in contact with the egg, several events must take place at the proper time in order for fertilization to take place. These include sperm penetration of the egg's cumulus cell layer, binding to the zona pellucida (the egg's protective coat), the sperm acrosome reaction (release of enzymes), penetration through the zona pellucida, and fusion of the sperm and egg plasma membranes.

The fertilized egg then progresses through the oviduct for another 72 hours and then enters the uterus. The egg undergoes several mitotic cycles during the first few days after fertilization, eventually forming a blastocyst. The blastocyst attaches to the uterine wall and then undergoes multiple steps to complete implantation. Human chorionic gonadotropin (hCG), a hormone released by the early embryo, is involved in events crucial to maintaining early pregnancy, including maintenance of the corpus luteum, which forms on the ovary after ovulation, progesterone production, and, perhaps implantation.

STRATEGIES FOR TARGET IDENTIFICATION

Recent advances in technology have provided new opportunities to use high-throughput methods[1] to address biological questions on a larger scale than was previously possible. This new approach to biomedical research represents a shift from the traditional, reductionist approach of

---

[1]Any approach using robotics, automated machines, and computers to process many samples at once.

BOX 2.1
Five Criteria Currently Used to Identify Functional Genes

The five criteria listed below are currently used to identify functional genes. Each has limitations and is likely to identify a different set of potential genes.

1. The presence of open reading frames (ORFs), which are strings of codons (nucleotide triplets encoding amino acids) bounded by start and stop signals.
2. Sequence features, in which genes exhibit nonrandom use of codons.
3. Sequence conservation among species.
4. Evidence for transcription, based on the identification of RNA or protein products (by use of microarrays, serial analysis of gene expression (SAGE), and transposon tagging, among other methods).
5. Gene inactivation, determined by blocking production of a functional protein through such techniques as RNA interference or gene disruption; a major drawback is redundancy, which precludes observation of a specific phenotype.

SOURCE: Snyder and Gerstein, 2003.

---

studying one or a very small number of molecules at a time to a larger-scale discovery or systems approach to studying hundreds or even thousands of molecules at once (Institute of Medicine, 2003).

For example, with the recent sequencing of entire genomes of many different species, there is now great interest in studying the products of all the genes encoded by the sequences. However, defining the genes[2] within a genome is not trivial. Most of an organism's DNA does not actually encode functional genes for proteins or other cellular components. Several approaches are used to identify functional genes (Box 2.1), but each has limitations and is likely to identify a different set of potential genes (Figure 2.5). These limitations are well known in model organisms such as yeast and are likely to be amplified in the more complex human genome (reviewed by Snyder and Gerstein, 2003). Thus, a variety of

---

[2]The definition of a "gene" has varied over time. A current definition is "a complete chromosomal segment responsible for making a functional product" (Snyder and Gerstein, 2003).

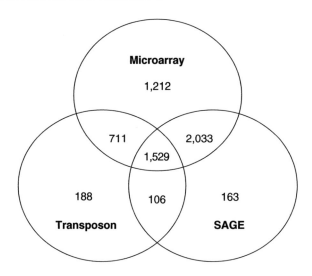

FIGURE 2.5 Functional genomics is best used in a combined fashion. Illustrated is the number of open reading frames in the yeast genome that were found to be transcribed based on data from microarray hybridization, SAGE, and transposon tagging experiments. Areas of overlap indicate that some transcripts were identified by more than one method.
SOURCE: Snyder and Gerstein, 2003.

approaches will be needed to identify and validate potential targets for contraceptive development. Some of these methods are described below.

Forward Gene Discovery

One method used to identify genes that are expressed in a particular cell or tissue type is the expressed sequence tag (EST) approach. This method entails sequencing many small nucleotide fragments, or tags, that have been derived from all the messenger RNAs (mRNAs) expressed in the given cell type. EST sequencing projects have provided publicly available information on more than 100,000 sequences for vertebrate reproductive tract tissues and cell types (e.g., ovary, testis, pituitary gland, oviduct, uterus, cervix, vagina, epididymis, prostate, gametes, and early embryos). These sequences are deposited in the public database at the National Center for Biotechnology Information[3] and are also assembled into clusters at

---

[3]See http://www.ncbi.nlm.nih.gov/.

UniGene.[4] Complementary DNA (cDNA) subtraction hybridization methods[5] and serial analysis of gene expression (SAGE) (Neilson et al., 2000), another method for global gene expression profiling, have also been useful to identify genes uniquely expressed in reproductive tissues (Neilson et al., 2000; Wang et al., 2001). *In silico* approaches, in which sequences already available in EST and SAGE databases are compared by using special computer programs to identify those that may be unique to a given tissue or cell type, can also be very powerful analytical methods. For example, several genes that are expressed exclusively in germ cells (Rajkovic et al., 2001) or epididymal tissues have been identified by this approach (Penttinen et al., 2003).

Because the ESTs are "tags," they are only a partial representation of the full-length mRNA. For transcripts that are long, short-lived, or in low abundance, the full-length mRNA and encoded proteins may be particularly difficult to identify. As a result, for a number of novel reproductive tract-specific transcripts, the full-length mRNA sequences and the protein products that they encode may still be unknown. This is problematic because many different mRNAs may be produced from a single gene via alternative splicing, transcription, or processing of the mRNA, and such alterations are known to result in gene transcripts that are unique to the testis (Kleene, 2001). Hence, full-length transcripts must be determined by complete sequencing of full-length cDNAs. Thus, in certain situations, more exhaustive analysis may be necessary for complete determination of the reproductive tract transcriptome and proteome.

The most extensive EST libraries of genes expressed in the male reproductive tract have been created by McCarrey and colleagues (McCarrey et al., 1999) and Ko and colleagues (Abe et al., 1998). These analyses were undertaken with mouse tissues because of the powerful genetics tools that are available for the mouse and the readily available source of material. Thus far, McCarrey and colleagues have sequenced 16,833 cDNA sequences. Additional sequencing is being done. In addition, the National Institutes of Health (NIH) Specialized Cooperative Centers Program in Reproduction Research has also sequenced alternative gene libraries and

---

[4]UniGene is an experimental system for automatically partitioning GenBank sequences into a nonredundant set of gene-oriented clusters. See http://www.ncbi.nlm.nih.gov/entrez/query.fcgi?db=unigene.

[5]A technique used to identify genes expressed differentially between two tissue samples. A large excess of mRNA from one sample is hybridized to cDNA from the other, and the double-stranded hybrids are removed by physical means. The remaining cDNAs are those that are not represented as RNA in the first sample and, thus, that are presumably expressed uniquely in the second sample. To improve specificity, the process is often repeated several times.

tissue sources.[6] Although serial analysis of gene expression has been conducted with human oocytes (Neilson et al., 2000), full-length sequences for most of the novel sequences and libraries of full-length sequences of human oocytes and early embryos are unavailable at present. Thus, projects to complete the determination of the novel reproductive tract-specific gene sequences of humans and model organisms, such as the mouse, are necessary and will need to include genomic and proteomic analysis of substitute nonhuman primate oocyte and early embryo cDNA libraries, similar to the exhaustive mouse sequence library analysis performed by Ko and colleagues (Ko et al., 2000).

Reverse Gene Discovery

One of the ways to identify and study gene function is to look for evidence of expression—that is, transcription of the gene into RNA. A recently developed technology, DNA microarrays,[7] provides a powerful, high-throughput method for studying transcription in specific cell types or tissues (Fodor et al., 1993; Schena et al., 1996). Microarrays have already been used to generate the data used in thousands of peer-reviewed publications and contributed to many public databases that are now used as research tools by the scientific community as a whole. This technology is widely thought to hold enormous potential for diverse applications, ranging from discovering new drug targets to identifying markers that could predict individual responses to drugs (reviewed by Chicurel and Dalma-Weiszhausz, 2002).

Microarrays that cover all known mouse genes as well as thousands of uncharacterized gene sequences are now being used to examine gene expression in numerous reproductive tissues, including the testis, ovary, and uterus of mice and humans (Borthwick et al., 2003; Burns et al., 2003; Carson et al., 2002; Giudice et al., 2002; Kao et al., 2002; Leo et al., 2001; McLean et al., 2002; reviewed by Schlecht and Primig, 2003; Schultz et al., 2003). Schultz and colleagues (2003) used microarray analyses of testicular cells to identify 351 mouse genes that appear to be sperm cell specific and that are expressed postmeiotically. The authors estimated that nearly 4 percent of the entire genome may be exclusively expressed in the male germ line. These genes thus represent a large number of germ cell-specific targets for contraceptive development. The databases containing the

---

[6]See http://www.nichd.nih.gov/about/cpr/rs/sccprr.htm (accessed August 2003).

[7]A DNA microarray consists of a glass microscope slide or silicon chip onto whose surface thousands of specific DNA sequences are spotted. Incubation with a labeled sample of nucleic acid such as mRNA can reveal which of the genes represented on the array are expressed in the sample and their relative levels.

mouse testis results are publicly available[8] and should be useful in the initial stages of developing a target for contraceptive development, although much work remains to characterize these genes and validate their potential as new targets for contraception.

Since the majority of these genes appear to be homologous (similar in sequence and function) and expressed in the human testis, new targets for potential contraceptive development can now be investigated. However, the field could be greatly advanced by the availability of standardized microarrays that include all genes, as well as alternatively spliced transcripts that are expressed in the reproductive tissues of humans and model organisms (e.g., mice). This would make it easier to compare the results among multiple investigators and would reduce the cost of such research. For example, efforts are ongoing to develop a microarray called EndoChip that represents gene expression during the window of implantation.[9]

Selective Gene Parsing

One can also discover putative genes of interest by identifying sequences that specify a particular function or location in the cell. For example, genes whose products function in specific cellular locations can be identified by searching for sequences that play an essential role in transporting proteins within the cell or in secreting proteins from a cell. Such proteins might facilitate communication between germ cells and their companion somatic cells or between germ cells or embryos and somatic cells of the reproductive tract.

One such approach, called a signal sequence trap (SST), has recently been used to identify mouse proteins that are either secreted by oocytes or in the oocyte cell membrane (Taft et al., 2002).[10] The SST methodology is based on the ability of a cloned sequence to drive the secretion of the yeast invertase enzyme, which is essential for the growth and survival of genetically modified yeast that are incapable of secreting this critical enzyme (Jacobs et al., 1997, 1999). When a piece of cDNA (derived from an oocyte, sperm cell, or other relevant reproductive tract cell) containing the appropriate signal peptide sequence is inserted in front of the yeast invertase gene, the ability of the enzyme-deficient yeast to secrete this critical enzyme is restored and the yeast can grow. The inserted cDNA

---

[8]See http://mrg.genetics.washington.edu/ (accessed July 2003).

[9]This work is funded by the NIH Reproductive Sciences Branch and the NIH Office of Research on Women's Health (Linda Giudice, personal communication, July 2003).

[10]John J. Eppig, The Jackson Laboratory, in a presentation at the International Symposium on New Frontiers in Contraceptive Research, Washington, DC, July 15-16, 2003.

can then be isolated from the growing yeast and the full-length cDNA containing this sequence can be identified.

Because these cDNAs encode putative ligands and receptors expressed by germ cells, embryos, or the reproductive tract, these regulators may serve as novel candidate targets for contraception. In theory, more extensive application of this approach to additional reproductive tract cells and tissues, including male germ cells or Sertoli cells or the epididymis, oviduct, cervix, or uterus, could lead to the identification of transmembrane and transport proteins that can be manipulated to produce a contraceptive effect. For example, tight junctions between the somatic Sertoli cells in the testis restrict the extracellular movement of molecules across the epithelium to the germinal cells on the luminal side. Little is known about the transport systems that deliver molecules to the protected compartment. Ion channels and transporter proteins may also be involved in sperm capacitation and fertilization.

In addition to targeting the transport systems themselves, one can even imagine exploiting the properties of the transport systems to specifically deliver contraceptives to testicular cells or other reproductive tract tissues, such as the uterus and prostate, that are also known to express many transporter proteins. Other approaches to selective gene parsing could potentially identify proteins with other functions that are amenable to modulation with drugs, including specific classes of enzymes such as kinases or phosphatases. For example, male germ-cell specific kinases have been identified (Nayak et al., 1998; Tanaka et al., 1999), but it is not certain that these are essential for spermatogenesis or sperm function, and at least some appear to be dispensable (Shinkai et al., 2002).

Proteomics

Most genes encode protein products, but RNA-based methods such as DNA arrays cannot precisely predict protein levels or protein modifications in a cell or tissue. Thus, many scientists are examining the expression, structure, and function of proteins directly. Much effort has recently been devoted to the study of proteomics, which attempts to define and analyze the entire protein complement (the proteome) involved in a particular biological process in a given cell, tissue, or organism. The challenges associated with proteomics research are enormous (Phizicky et al., 2003; Sali et al., 2003; reviewed by Tyers and Mann, 2003). Many different proteins can be produced from a single gene because of such regulatory events as alternate splicing of the mRNA as well as biochemical modifications to the resultant protein, including glycosylation, acetylation, phosphorylation, and proteolytic processing. An individual's proteome can change over time, depending on a whole host of variables, including stage of development, exposure to external factors, and the state of health or disease.

Furthermore, despite recent technological advances, current methods, instrumentation, and information technologies are still far from optimal; and many obstacles remain to the effective and efficient achievement of the goals of proteomics research (Boguski and McIntosh, 2003; Phizicky et al., 2003; Tyers and Mann, 2003; Vidal, 2001). For instance, additional high-throughput technologies and new computational methods to analyze the resultant large data sets are needed. The incorporation of medical informatics will also be critical, since clinical application of proteomics will increasingly require the integrated analysis of genetic, cellular, molecular, and clinical information and the expertise of pathologists, epidemiologists, and biostatisticians.

The plethora of information generated also poses challenges for data management. There is a great need for databases that use agreed-upon standards for protein data to facilitate comparisons and integration of complex and disparate kinds of protein information into a biological atlas. Because the current principal protein databases[11] emphasize molecular and cellular features and annotation, they are not well suited to represent physiology, and there is currently no reliable way to retrieve groups of proteins based on well-known pathways or functional classifications (Boguski and McIntosh, 2003). In addition, public access to the raw data is essential so that the numerous individuals working across the many fields of biomedical research can participate in the research. The proteomics community will need to work closely with scientists focused on biological problems to translate the broad but shallow proteomic data into deeper understanding of proteomics. One step in that direction has been taken by the Human Proteome Organization and the European Bioinformatics Institute, which together have started the Proteomics Standard Initiative[12] to exchange protein–protein interaction data and other proteomic data.

Access to the technologies needed to study proteomics may also be limited by their cost, so there is much interest in facilitating more widespread use of tools for proteomics research. At the same time, it is important to coordinate large-scale research efforts in proteomics both to avoid duplication and to provide strong rationale for funding agencies. One practical bottleneck to these approaches—and in fact, to most large-scale, systematic research projects—has been the limited availability of validated

---

[11]Collections of protein sequences date back to the 1960s, preceding GenBank by nearly 20 years. Since the early 1990s, important utilitarian goals of protein databases have included minimal redundancy, maximal annotation, and integration with other databases. These principles continue to be stressed today (see Boguski and McIntosh, 2003).

[12]See http://psidev.sourceforge.net/ (accessed October 2003).

genome-wide cDNA for use in the capture of protein complexes (Tyers and Mann, 2003). The FlexGene consortium[13] between academic institutions and industry aims to develop complete cDNA collections for use by the biomedical community.

A variety of other technical challenges also limit the quality and usefulness of data generated by proteomics research. Meaningful interpretation of results depends upon careful study design and high-quality[14] biological samples; but fundamental challenges involving biological variability, preanalytic factors,[15] and analytical reproducibility remain to be resolved (reviewed by Boguski and McIntosh, 2003). For instance, in the case of human proteomics, sample materials may be limited and of inconsistent quality because of protein degradation or variability in collection, handling, and storage procedures. In addition, most gene expression and proteomic analyses involving human specimens will be observational studies out of necessity, leading to important questions about possible biases and confounding factors in the populations from which the samples are drawn. Indeed, in referring to functional genomics technologies and their relevance in clinical medicine, Margolin (2001) has admonished that "Scientists . . . need to avoid the tendency, often driven by the high price of some of the newer techniques, of running under-controlled experiments or experiments with fewer repeated conditions than would have been accepted with standard techniques" (p. 234). Boguski and McIntosh (2003) note that the same caveat applies to proteomics research, but perhaps even more so because a framework to estimate appropriate sample sizes has yet to be determined and the nature of the technology creates substantial challenges to progress in achieving this goal.

Despite these current limitations, scientists have great hope for the potential benefits of proteomics research. Moreover, drug discovery and development could benefit greatly from the new information generated (Hanash, 2003; Pawson and Nash, 2003; Tyers and Mann, 2003; Vidal, 2001). Because most drugs target proteins, it is likely that proteomics will

---

[13]See http://www.hip.harvard.edu/ (accessed October 2003).

[14]Two issues associated with specimens of almost any kind are sample quality and number. Quality involves both the preservation of molecular features (such as intact and representative proteins) and the assurance of both inter- and intrasample homogeneity (Boguski and McIntosh, 2003).

[15]These refer to those factors, both known and unknown, that may be present in a subject or that may arise in any of the steps before a laboratory test and data analysis. Examples include genotype; physiological attributes such as age, gender, reproductive status, lifestyle effects (for example, diet or smoking), and drugs taken; and specimen collection, handling, and processing protocols. Uncontrollable variables must be well understood to be able to separate their effects from the object or process under study. Most errors in clinical laboratory tests are known to occur in the preanalytical phase (Boguski and McIntosh, 2003).

play a major role in future drug discovery, development, and clinical application, provided that suitable platforms become available.

The proteomics approach is already being used to identify potential new targets for contraceptives. John Herr and colleagues at the University of Virginia have been analyzing human sperm and mouse eggs using tandem mass spectrometry (a method for separating molecular and atomic particles by mass) to determine what proteins exist in these cells, the relative abundance of individual proteins, and their unique properties.[16] The objective of these analyses is to identify, clone, and characterize novel proteins that may be targets for drug-based contraceptives or that could potentially be used to make contraceptive vaccines (which would induce an immune response against proteins specific to the reproductive process and therefore block fertility). The databases created by these studies are referred to as the Human Sperm Proteome and the Mouse Egg Proteome. Similarly, the lists of proteins identified in each cell type are catalogued in the Sperm Protein Encyclopedia and the Egg Protein Encyclopedia. The former currently contains approximately 2000 proteins, of which 850 have been sequenced and 78 are novel or uncharacterized. About 280 proteins in the latter database have been sequenced and 32 are novel or uncharacterized.[17]

To identify new candidates as targets for drug-based contraceptives, the group has examined key chemical modifications (phosphorylation) of regulatory proteins and the enzymes that catalyze those modifications (known as kinases). To optimize the identification of proteins that could potentially be useful for contraceptive vaccine production, the group has also focused on proteins that are found on the surfaces of sperm and eggs and on proteins that have already been found to induce antibody production in the serum of infertile men and women.

Lipidomics

The process of reproduction involves multiple events in which membranes of different cells come into intimate contact, including interactions of male germ cells with Sertoli cells, the binding of sperm to the cells lining the oviduct, the fusion of the sperm and the egg, the attachment of the embryo to the cells lining the uterus, and the formation of the placenta. While these interactions may involve proteins on the surface of the opposing cells, the lipid structures of the cell membrane in which the proteins

---

[16]John C. Herr, Professor of Cell Biology at the University of Virginia, in a presentation at the International Symposium on New Frontiers in Contraceptive Research, Washington, DC, July 15-16, 2003.
[17]Personal communication with John C. Herr, November 2003.

are embedded may also play key roles and are therefore potential targets for contraceptives. In addition, physiological processes occurring in germ cells may involve changes in membrane lipid composition that alter membrane structure or trigger signaling cascades. For example, sperm membranes have cholesterol-rich areas, and the removal of cholesterol from the sperm membranes is involved in triggering sperm capacitation (Davis, 1976, 1980, 1981; Travis and Kopf, 2002). Changes in cholesterol occur during the natural process of sperm activation in the vagina or can be induced by incubation of sperm with cholesterol-binding substances (e.g., albumin and cyclodextrins). Signaling molecules, including a variety of receptors, are localized in specialized membrane domains called rafts. Modulation of the lipid contents of these domains is known to alter protein function. A number of proteins are tethered to membranes by a phospholipid called phosphatidylinositol or as a result of posttranslational modifications with fatty acids, cholesterol, or intermediates in the cholesterol synthesis pathway. The integrity of cell membranes is critical to cell survival. Agents (e.g., detergents and surfactants) that disrupt the membrane lipid structure are well known to be spermicidal and are widely used as contraceptives (Bernstein, 1974), but they also have effects on non-germ cell membranes (e.g., the cells lining the reproductive tract). Finally, the entry of certain microorganisms into cells involves fusion with or uptake by the membrane, and therefore, entry into the cell is potentially sensitive to agents that affect lipid composition and membrane structure–function.

The lipid components of membranes that are of particular interest include sterols, glycolipids, and ether lipids. Evidence from functional genomics experiments with mice has suggested important roles for lipid metabolism in male germ cell function. Spermatogenesis is severely impaired in mice lacking seminolipid, the major glycolipid of mature mammalian sperm (Fujimoto et al., 2000; Honke et al., 2002). Mice that lack the genes for some of the enzymes required in the synthesis of specific types of lipids also have impaired fertility. For example, targeted deletion of the ganglioside synthase gene in mice, which results in deficiencies in all gangliosides (a class of lipid), is associated with azoospermia and male infertility (Takamiya et al., 1998). Mutation of another gene involved in the synthesis of ether lipids (also known as plasmalogens) is also associated with male infertility (Rodemer et al., 2003), as is inactivation of the hormone-sensitive lipase gene, which encodes an enzyme that hydrolyzes cholesterol esters and triglycerides (Chung et al., 2001; Osuga et al., 2000). Data linking lipid function to female fertility are more limited, but at least one mouse model implicates such a link. Female mice lacking the scavenger receptor involved in the uptake of high-density lipoprotein cholesterol are infertile (Trigatti et al., 1999).

Other types of experiments have also suggested a role for lipids in fertility. For instance, an inhibitor of the enzyme involved in the transfer of glucose to a type of lipid known as ceramide causes reversible infertility in male mice without significant side effects (van der Spoel et al., 2002). Sperm-immobilizing antibodies that react with seminolipid have been described as well (Tsuji et al., 1992).

The lipid content and composition of the testis and male reproductive tract and the cholesterol-rich domains of sperm have been the most studied, but very little effort has been made to examine the lipid content and composition of the oocyte or cells of the female reproductive tract. Human tissues may contain more than 1,000 major lipids, including classes such as glycolipids, sterols, and phospholipids, as well as an unknown number of less prevalent minor species (Wilson, 2003). Quantifying and analyzing the lipid components of cells is thus a complex undertaking, but advances in technologies such as mass spectrometry and liquid chromatography are emerging that can increase the speed and scope of such research. Efforts are also under way to identify and characterize the multitude of enzymes that synthesize and modulate lipids.

Characterization of the lipid composition of reproductive cells, including any novel lipid structures and the biosynthetic pathways by which they are generated, could reveal opportunities for contraceptive targets, such as interference of sperm–egg membrane fusion or premature activation of sperm, which would result in a contraceptive effect. A chemical genetics screen to discover agents that selectively act on and disrupt gamete membrane lipid domains is one possible exercise that could be fruitful for identification of new contraceptives.

Lipids also play important signaling roles in reproduction. For example, platelet-activating factor, an acetylated glycerophospholipid, has been shown to be involved in several reproductive processes, including ovarian, uterine, and oviductal function (Harper, 1989; Ishii et al., 2002; Ishii and Shimizu, 2000; Logan and Roudebush, 2000; Toledo et al., 2003). It causes activation of sperm and oocytes by inducing influx of extracellular calcium. Prostaglandin signaling plays a role in the implantation process. Mice deficient in the COX-2 cyclooxygenase (COX) display abnormalities in the implantation process, particularly the early decidual response (Lim et al., 1997). Evidence suggestive of a role of prostaglandins in the human implantation process includes the presence of COX-1 and COX-2 in the human endometrium, mainly the glandular epithelium, during the presumptive implantation period (Marions et al., 1999) and from an examination of prenatal use of nonsteroidal anti-inflammatory drugs (NSAIDs), drugs that inhibit COX enzymes, that indicated an increased risk of miscarriage in users of aspirin and other NSAIDs (Li et al., 2003). One of the key prostaglandins involved in implantation is thought to be prostacyclin, a ligand for peroxisome proliferator-activated receptor delta, a member of the nuclear receptor family expressed in subluminal stromal cells in the rodent uterus (Ding et al., 2003; Lim and Dey, 2002). The transcription factor peroxisome proliferator-activated receptor delta is implicated in the implantation process (Lim and Dey, 2000; Matsumoto et al., 2001). Another lipid implicated in implantation is the endocannabinoid anandamide,[18] a ligand for the cannabinoid receptors CB1-R and CB2-R (Habayeb et al., 2002; Paria and Dey, 2000; Paria et al., 2002), which are expressed in the preimplantation embryo and in the reproductive tract (CB1-R only). Uterine anandamide levels in the mouse are reduced at the time of implantation and are highest at interimplantation sites. Endocannabinoids at low levels accelerate trophoblast[19] differentiation, but at high levels they inhibit trophoblast differentiation and arrest embryo development. Natural and synthetic agonists of the cannabinoid receptors have similar effects. Thus, it has been postulated that endocannabinoids play an important role in controlling the synchrony of embryo development for implantation in rodents. Anandamide is present in human reproductive tract fluids (Schuel et al., 2002), and high anandamide levels are associated with failures of in vitro fertilization (Maccarrone et al., 2002).

Glycomics

Scientists estimate that 50-80 percent of proteins contain glycan[20] structures, and these structures can play an important role in cell interactions and signaling. The potential role of glycobiology in contraceptive development is based on the evidence that specific glycan structures are involved in gamete maturation, function, sperm–reproductive tract interactions, and sperm–egg binding.[21] The evidence supporting a role for glycans in sperm–egg binding, as well as the interaction of gametes with the cells lining the male and female reproductive tracts, has been described in the literature for many decades; however, there is still debate about the exact components and mechanisms of the interaction (Primakoff and Myles, 2002; Talbot et al., 2003; reviewed by Wassarman, 2002). It is well

---

[18]Anandamide, also known as arichidonylethanolamide, is derived from arachidonate an essential fatty acid that humans use to synthesize regulatory molecules such as prostaglandins and thromboxanes. It is also referred to as an endocannabinoid due to its ability to bind cannabinoid receptors.

[19]The part of the early embryo that attaches to the wall of the uterus.

[20]Any of many carbohydrates that are made up of chains of simple sugars.

[21]This section is based largely on written input provided by Diana Blithe, Ph.D., Contraception and Reproductive Health Branch NICHD, NIH, DHHS.

accepted that protein glycosylation[22] is involved in these processes, and this assumption has been used as the basis for the theoretical development of contraceptive agents. As noted above, glycolipids play important roles in spermatogenesis as well. However, contraceptive product development has been slow because of difficulties in precisely analyzing the glycan structures involved and because gamete glycosylation is species specific, which likely contributes to the inhibition of cross-species fertilization. Advances in recombinant DNA technology have not simplified matters because the resultant recombinant proteins often do not contain native glycan structures. However, new technologies, such as carbohydrate microarrays (Service, 2003), that could speed research progress and scope in this field are beginning to emerge. Similarly, technical advances that have improved the sensitivities of existing analytical techniques, such as mass spectrometry and nuclear magnetic resonance, have made it easier to characterize sugars from much smaller amounts of sample material. Moreover, the National Institute of General Medical Sciences at NIH has recently provided funding for the development of tools and resources for glycomics research through a "glue grant"—a funding mechanism that supports large-scale collaborative efforts with the goal of addressing problems beyond the reach of individual investigators. One of the many goals of the Consortium for Functional Glycomics is to determine glycan profiles of mouse and human tissues, cells, and proteins, including the testis and ovary. Research tools such as arrays and mice with gene knockouts for enzymes that add or modify carbohydrate structures on proteins are being made available to scientists through core facilities.[23]

Potential glycan targets for contraception include immunogenic molecules on the sperm surface that could be used to inhibit sperm motility in the reproductive tract, the enzymatic activity associated with sperm penetration of the cell layer surrounding the egg, or binding of the sperm to the egg. In addition, there is potential to interfere with cellular interactions during gamete maturation so that the appropriate glycans are not present on the mature gametes or the gametes fail to fully mature. In either case, function would be impaired.

Specific glycan structures are generated on sperm surfaces by selective processing in the testis, or are added during maturation as sperm pass through the epididymis, or during activation in the female reproductive tract (Srivastav, 2000). One glycan in particular appears to be required for interaction between maturing sperm and cells of the testis (Akama et

---

[22]The addition of a chain of sugars to a protein in order to make a glycoprotein.
[23]See http://web.mit.edu/glycomics/consortium/ (accessed November 2003).

al., 2002; Muramatsu, 2002). Production of a mouse in which the enzyme required for the formation of this glycan structure is knocked out leads to sterile male mice but fertile females (Akama et al., 2002). In another study, inhibitors of glycoprocessing enzymes were used to induce reversible sterility in male mice with no other apparent phenotypic effects. Female mice treated with the inhibitors had normal fertility (van der Spoel et al., 2002). The latter study was unable to determine whether the effects of the inhibitors were on glycoproteins or glycolipids, or both. Nonetheless, the ability to deliver an agent to the testis, as well as the apparent testis specificity of the impact, makes these targets appealing for contraceptive development.

A number of proteins are inserted into the sperm membrane as sperm progress through the testis and epididymis. One protein, an immunogenic structure called sperm agglutination antigen 1 (SAGA-1), is a membrane-anchored[24] glycoprotein that is acquired in the epididymis and that is localized over the entire head of sperm. The protein core of this molecule is found on lymphocytes (a type of white blood cell) and sperm; however, the carbohydrate-specific portion of the molecule is found only on sperm, thus making it an attractive target for contraception (McCauley et al., 2002).

Glycan structures on a given protein are often tissue-specific. One such molecule is glycodelin. Glycodelin has two differently glycosylated forms, one secreted by uterine endometrium in the female reproductive tract (GdA) and the other secreted by seminal vesicle cells in the male reproductive tract (GdS). Unique glycosylation of GdA versus GdS determines inhibitory activity in sperm–egg binding. GdA inhibits sperm–egg binding and is secreted into uterine fluid beginning about 4 days after ovulation. In contrast, GdS does not interfere with sperm–egg binding (reviewed by Halttunen et al., 2000).

Sperm–egg binding is a carbohydrate-mediated event. A zona pellucida protein known as ZP3 is believed to be a ligand for sperm binding to the zona pellucida of the egg (Primakoff and Myles, 2002; Talbot et al., 2003; reviewed by Wassarman, 2002). Glycans present on ZP3 have been implicated in the binding of sperm. Early experiments suggested that an enzyme present on sperm could bind to oligosaccharide residues on ZP3 (Talbot et al., 2003). Evidence also indicates that activated eggs lack the oligosaccharide structure that is the proposed binding target for sperm, thus protecting against fertilization by more than one sperm (Koyanagi and Honegger, 2003; Vo et al., 2003).

---

[24]Via a glycosylphosphatidylinositol (GPI) membrane anchor. For more detail please see the section on sperm-egg interaction.

The species specificity of glycosylation remains an important issue in studies of protein function. Although ZP3 is widely accepted as the sperm receptor, the actual glycan structures involved have not been characterized. Substitution of human ZP3 in a mouse ZP3 knockout resulted in restoration of fertility in the female, but specificity for mouse sperm rather than for human sperm was retained (Rankin et al., 1998). The presumption is that human ZP3 was appropriately glycosylated by the mouse glycoprocessing machinery to provide species-specific binding. However, the potential functional impact of species-specificity or tissue specificity of glycosylation is often overlooked when recombinant technology is used to produce proteins (see Chapter 3 for more detail). For example, glycosylation of recombinant ZP3 is required for functional capability (Gahlay and Gupta, 2003). Sperm incubated with recombinant glycosylated ZP3 could undergo the acrosomal reaction but sperm incubated with unglycosylated ZP3 made in *E. coli* could not undergo the reaction. In some cases, not only the presence of glycosylation but also the specific components of the glycan are critical. For instance, GdA synthesized in cultured human kidney cells retained the ability to inhibit sperm–egg binding, but this function was lost when GdA was produced in cultured hamster ovary cells (Van den Nieuwenhof et al., 2000).

Thus, despite the consensus that glycans are obligatory for sperm–egg interaction, the lack of knowledge about the specific structural components involved has hampered contraceptive development based on the egg as a target. Identification of the precise structure of the critical glycans on both the human egg and sperm will be necessary to plan an effective contraceptive strategy based on glycobiology.

Deciphering Cell Regulatory Networks

Protein Networks

To truly understand how cells work at the molecular level, one must know not only what proteins are present but also how they function and interact with each other in a cellular context. Conversely, identifying the interacting partners of proteins is very helpful in deducing protein function, as proteins that interact with one another or that are part of the same protein complex are generally involved in the same cellular processes.

Structured ensembles of proteins and other molecules perform many vital cellular functions. Frequently, these protein complexes comprise 10 or more components (Sali et al., 2003). Small portions of proteins, known as interaction domains, mediate and regulate protein complex formation. Cells use a limited set of interaction domains, which are joined together in diverse combinations, to direct the actions of protein networks. Interaction domains are remarkably versatile in their binding properties, as individual domains can engage several distinct targets, either simultaneously or at successive stages of signaling. Different members of the same domain type can also bind to quite different targets. Regulation of protein complex formation frequently depends on biochemical modifications of the interaction domains, including phosphorylation, hydroxylation, acetylation, methylation, and ubiquitination (Pawson and Nash, 2003). Interaction domains play a pervasive role in regulating the dynamic organization and function of cells. For example, these domains mediate the association of cell surface receptors with their targets; the formation of signaling protein complexes inside the cell; and protein movement, organization, function, and degradation within the cell. Moreover, protein interaction domains not only enable linear pathways but can also generate more complex networks that facilitate cross talk between pathways and that integrate signals from distinct sources (reviewed by Pawson and Nash, 2003).

The Protein Quaternary Structure (PQS)[25] database currently contains ~10,000 structurally defined protein assemblies of presumed biological significance derived from a variety of organisms. It is very difficult to predict the potential number of different protein complexes with unique structures and biological functions, especially in complicated organisms such as humans. The calculation of such estimates is a formidable task because of the many possible components and the various life spans of the protein complexes (transient versus stable complexes). In addition, there is no obvious definition of a "protein complex" and no means to determine whether two protein complexes are of different types. However, currently available data suggest that there are at least 30,000 protein–protein interactions in yeast, a simple model organism. This number corresponds to about nine partners per protein, but these are not all necessarily direct or occurring at the same time. The human proteome may have an order of magnitude more protein complexes than the yeast cell (reviewed by Sali et al., 2003).

By studying protein complexes, it is possible in principle to assemble an atlas of protein networks within a cell. A variety of experimental methods are available for the identification and characterization of protein complexes, and each has different advantages and limitations (Box 2.2 and Table 2.1). Two of the most commonly used techniques for identifying protein complexes are: the two-hybrid system to detect binary protein interactions in cells; and biochemical purification of protein complexes followed by protein identification by mass spectrometry. Such approaches have been used to identify proteins that interact with an oocyte-specific

---

[25]See http://pqs.ebi.ac.uk/pqs-doc.shtml (accessed July 2003).

BOX 2.2
Experimental Methods for
Structural Characterization of Assemblies

A variety of methods are available for the experimental determination of protein complex structure. These are described below.

X-ray crystallography is the most powerful method for structure determination because it is capable of providing an atomic structure of the whole assembly. When suitable crystals and high-resolution crystallographic data are obtained, there is little need for other methods of structure characterization.

Nuclear magnetic resonance (NMR) spectroscopy allows determination of molecular structures of increasingly large subunits and even their complexes. Although NMR analysis is generally not as applicable as X-ray crystallography to protein structures with more than 300 amino acid residues, it can be applied to molecules in solution and is more suitable than X-ray crystallography for study of their dynamics and interactions in solution.

Electron crystallography (two-dimensional electron microscopy, or 2D EM) and single-particle analysis can reveal the shape and symmetry of an assembly, sometimes at resolutions near the atomic level but more frequently at an intermediate resolution. Segmentation of the electron density may lead to an approximate configuration of the subunits in a complex. Proteins whose structures are already known can then be fitted into these density maps with an accuracy approaching 1/10 the resolution of the EM reconstruction.

Electron tomography is based on multiple tilted views of the same object. Although it can be used to study the structures of isolated macromolecular assemblies at a relatively low resolution, its true potential lies in visualizing the assemblies in an unperturbed cellular context.

Immunoelectron microscopy can be used to determine the approximate position of a protein in the context of an assembly. This task is achieved by using a construct of the protein of interest that binds to a gold-labeled antibody. The relative position of the gold particles is then identified by electron microscopy.

Chemical cross-linking with mass spectroscopy can be used to identify binary and higher-order protein contacts. The approach relies on bi- and trifunctional cross-linking reagents that covalently link proteins interacting with each other. Proteolytic digestion and subsequent mass spectroscopic identification of the cross-linked species reveal their composition. In addition, chemical cross-linking of specific residue types has recently been used to obtain intramolecular distance restraints.

Affinity purification with mass spectroscopy combines purification of protein complexes with identification of their individual components by mass spectroscopy. During cell lysis, the whole assembly is partially broken into smaller complexes that are then isolated by a variety of methods, such as those relying on fusion proteins or antibodies as baits for affinity purification. The subunits in these smaller complexes are usually identified by a combination of gel electrophoresis and mass spectroscopy.

Fluorescence resonance energy transfer (FRET) occurs when a higher-energy fluorophore stimulates emission by a lower-energy fluorophore that is within ~60 Å of its inducer. It can be applied to monitor protein interactions if one protein is fused to a fluorescence donor and its potential partner is fused to a fluorescence acceptor. Fluorescence donors and acceptors are usually spectral derivatives of the green fluorescence protein.

Site-directed mutagenesis and a variety of biochemical experiments (for example, footprinting) can reveal which subunits in a complex interact with each other and sometimes what face is involved in the interaction.

Yeast two-hybrid system detects binary protein interactions by activating expression of a reporter gene upon direct binding between the two proteins being tested. The approach is based on the modularity of transcription factors that consist of a DNA-binding domain and an activation domain, each of which is fused to two different genes encoding the proteins whose interaction is tested. If the two fusion proteins expressed are in contact with each other, the two modules of the transcription factor are united, thereby inducing transcription of a set of reporter genes. Expression of the reporter genes, in turn, is easily detected by a variety of tests, such as yeast colony color and ability to grow in nutrient-deficient media. The method is suitable for high-throughput applications.

Protein arrays immobilize a variety of bait proteins, such as antibodies and glutathione *S*-transferase, onto an array on a specially treated surface; the array is then probed with sample proteins, resulting in the detection of binary interactions. mRNA expression arrays immobilize stretches of mRNA and are used to measure the concentration of mRNA species in a sample as a function of tissue type, cell cycle, and other environmental conditions. Such data sets have been used to detect functionally linked proteins, which include proteins whose expression is coregulated because they are members of the same assembly, are encoded on the same operon, or belong to the same biochemical pathway.

SOURCE: Sali et al., 2003; see also Table 2.1.

TABLE 2.1 Experimental and Theoretical Methods That Can Provide Information About the Structure of a Protein Complex Structure

Type	Subunit structure	Subunit shape	Subunit-subunit contact	Subunit proximity	Subunit stochiometry	Assembly symmetry	Assembly shape	Assembly structure
X-ray crystallography	✓	✓	✓	✓	✓	✓	✓	✓
NMR spectroscopy	✓	✓	✓	✓	✓	✓	✓	✓
2D and single-particle electron microscopy	✓	✓	✓	✓		✓	✓	
Electron tomography	✓	✓	✓	✓		✓	✓	
Immuno-electron microscopy			✓	✓		✓		
Chemical cross-linking	✓		✓	✓				
Affinity purification mass spectroscopy								
Fluorescence resonance energy transfer (FRET)			✓	✓				
Site-directed mutagenesis			✓					
Yeast two-hybrid system			✓					
Protein arrays		✓	✓					
Protein structure prediction	✓							
Computational docking			✓					
Bioinformatics			✓					

NOTE: The annotations below each of the panels list the aspects of an assembly that might be obtained by the corresponding method. Subunit-subunit contact indicates knowledge about protein pairs that are in contact with each other, and in some cases about the face that is involved in the contact. Subunit proximity indicates whether two proteins are close to each other relative to the size of the assembly, but not necessarily whether they are in direct contact. Subunit stochiometry indicates the number of subunits of a given type that occur in the assembly. Assembly symmetry indicates the symmetry of the arrangement of the subunits in the assembly. Gray boxes indicate extreme difficulty in obtaining the corresponding information by a given method. (See also Box 2.2.)
SOURCE: Adapted from Sali et al., 2003.

enzyme that functions in a key protein degradation pathway (Suzumori et al., 2003). With advances in automated technologies, protein interactions can now also be identified through a variety of high-throughput screening tests, but predictive data must still be validated by direct analysis of protein complexes from cells. Individually, each approach is prone to error and fails to capture all the relevant information about the dynamic activities of proteins within cells, but, taken together, they provide a higher level of information. For example, combining the results of several techniques has identified an interaction network in yeast (reviewed by Pawson and Nash, 2003). The protein complexes of this network can now be tested by both biochemical and genetic means.

The expectation is that understanding the network of cellular protein interactions will allow scientists to investigate proteins of interest in greater detail and in ways that are not currently possible. Moreover, the modulation of protein interactions is a promising approach to drug design because small molecules (e.g., kinase and phosphatase inhibitors) can be used to modify protein complexes in a variety of ways. The direct approach of inhibiting interactions is potentially of great value and has already yielded some potential drug compounds with in vivo activity for therapeutic indications (Cochran, 2000).

Genetic Networks

Recent experiments using the techniques described in this chapter have generated data that can be used to ascertain the functions of many genes. A major challenge that remains is the development of a fundamental description of cellular function at the DNA level by determining the complex dynamic interactions and regulation of all the genes of an organism—its genetic networks (Banerjee and Zhang, 2002; Hasty et al., 2001). Genetic networks are models of how external signals affect gene expression and how changing activity of one gene or a group of genes affects the activity of other genes (Brazhnik et al., 2002). The goal is to link the genes and their products into functional pathways, circuits, and networks. Models of gene regulation commonly represent networks of genes as if they directly affect each other. Although genes do not interact directly with other genes, network models use this concept because gene induction or repression occurs through the actions of specific proteins, which are, in turn, products of other genes. The theoretical concept of interacting genetic networks was first explored nearly 30 years ago, but progress in the field had to await technological advances that could facilitate the collection of data on gene expression and function on a larger scale (Hasty et al., 2001).

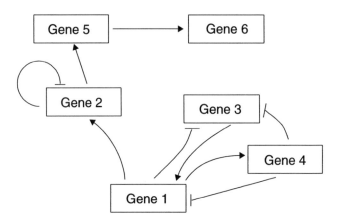

FIGURE 2.6 An example of a hypothetical gene network. Lines show direct effects, with arrows indicating activation and bars indicating inhibition.

Models of genetic networks are commonly represented by diagrams (Figure 2.6) that display causal relationships between gene activities (Brazhnik et al., 2002). These schematics of genetic networks resemble circuit diagrams, and in many ways this analogy highlights the motivation for a quantitative description of gene regulation. If a genetic network were a complex electrical circuit, there would be an accompanying set of equations that would reliably describe its functionality. This description would be built from knowledge of the properties of the individual gene components (analogous to resistors, capacitors, inductors, and so on) and provide a framework for predicting the behavior that would result from modifications in the circuit (Hasty et al., 2001). Currently, though, it is quite difficult to simplify complex genetic networks into a set of equations.

Research on genetic networks has two major goals: first, to understand the dynamics and design principles of gene regulation and, second, to reverse engineer genetic networks from experimental measurements (Brazhnik et al., 2002). In recent years, the majority of research in genetic networks has focused on methodologies for reconstructing genetic networks from experimental observations of gene expression, presumably because of the abundance of microarray data. However, many interactions between genes have also been discovered through traditional molecular biology approaches. Genetic networks can be postulated by combining data about these interactions from various sources. The GeNet database[26] is an example of an electronic repository for such information. Experimental techniques alone are limited in their ability to deduce genetic networks. Similarly, although computational models can offer insight into basic mechanisms, modeling must ultimately be connected to experimental systems so that verifiable predictions can be made. The most useful methods will likely entail a combination of novel experimental approaches and new computational modeling techniques (Hasty et al., 2001). Thus, it is necessary to develop sophisticated computational tools to extract relevant information from different data sources (van Someren et al., 2002). Many different approaches for developing models of genetic networks have been proposed and tested, and each of the modeling techniques has its own merits and drawbacks (Brazhnik et al., 2002; Hasty et al., 2001). Examples of methods used to decipher gene expression data are described in Box 2.3.

So far, few computational modeling studies have involved tight coupling between modeling and experiments (Hasty et al., 2001). Additionally, current experimental data from which networks are inferred can be extremely difficult to analyze and interpret because of inconsistencies from one experiment to the next. Furthermore, in the foreseeable future, the numbers of samples and data points, even in the largest experiments, do not provide enough information to construct a full, detailed model with high statistical confidence. Thus, the results of many more experiments will be needed to develop genetic networks with high degrees of accuracy and predictability. Compounding these issues is a great need to integrate diverse data types and to construct tools that will assimilate the information into biological models (Banerjee and Zhang, 2002).

Defining genetic networks may be one of the most challenging tasks of functional genomics. However, when successful, understanding the network of regulatory interactions could yield a wealth of useful information, such as the pathway to which a gene belongs, the function of the gene in terms of how it influences other genes, and the identification of genes that serve as pathway initiators and that are therefore potential drug targets (van Someren et al., 2002). For example, genetic networks might allow genes to be ranked according to their importance in controlling and regulating cellular events. In this way, knowledge about genetic networks might provide valuable information for drug discovery and development by aiding the prioritization of targets (Brazhnik et al., 2002).

---

[26]GeNet contains information on the functional organization of regulatory genes networks acting at embryogenesis. See http://www.csa.ru/Inst/gorb_dep/inbios/genet/genet.htm (accessed October 2003).

BOX 2.3
Examples of Methods Proposed for Inferring Gene Networks
from Experimental mRNA Expression Data

Boolean method: The Boolean method is a popular method for analysis of gene expression data that assumes that genes with similar expression patterns are functionally related to each other ("clustering algorithms"). Although in widespread use, this method has severe limitations in deciphering gene networks, especially complex, heavily connected networks. Other methods based on more sophisticated statistical analyses also exist, but in general, the correlation is not sufficient to infer causality between genes. Several methods rely on a simplification in which genes are considered to be expressed either at a fixed rate or not at all. These approaches suffer from an inability to capture intermediate levels of gene expression and can easily generate spurious results.

Linear method: More challenging but potentially more accurate representations of gene networks use continuous functions in which expression levels are allowed to take any positive value. These approaches are mathematically implemented by difference or differential equations, either linear or nonlinear.

Nonlinear kinetic method: More realistic, but also more difficult, approaches use nonlinear kinetics to represent the rate of transcription, such as neural network-like functions similar to those of enzyme kinetics. Their use is hindered by their requirement for larger amounts of data.

SOURCE: Brazhnik et al., 2002.

TARGET VALIDATION STUDIES

Model Organisms as a Necessary Step in the
Development of Future Contraceptives

Genetic screens can be conducted with a variety of model organisms, including mice, fish, frogs, worms, and flies.[27] Both forward genetic screens (those that identify a gene on the basis of phenotype [e.g., infertil-

---

[27]Examples of screens in each of these model organisms were presented at the International Symposium on New Frontiers in Contraceptive Research, Washington, DC, July 15-16, 2003.

ity]) and reverse genetic screens (those that block a function of a reproductive tract-specific gene via gene knockout or knockdown approaches with the goal of defining the function of a gene in reproduction) are extremely valuable and complementary. These in vivo genetic screens are key steps in the validation process. Flies, fish, worms, and mice are the easiest in vivo models to manipulate for contraceptive evaluation. The mouse has been an important mammalian model for understanding and studying reproduction in humans for many years because most of the reproductive hormones and growth factors are highly conserved between mice and humans. However, target validation in mice or lower organisms is not foolproof. For example, targeting a particular gene may inhibit fertility in mice but not humans, or vice versa, because of gene redundancy, a situation in which multiple genes within a genome can perform a similar function in a given biological process or pathway.

Reverse Genetics

The target discovery experiments described in the first part of this chapter will likely identify hundreds of candidate targets for follow-up studies. In most cases, the next step is to undertake reverse genetic studies with mammals. Experimental approaches include "knockout" models, in which a specific gene is deleted or rendered nonfunctional in animals, and "knockdown" models, in which the level of expression of a particular gene is reduced. Knockdown approaches that use RNA interference techniques (described below) have been successful in the analysis of a few genes expressed by oocytes. Other knockdown approaches include RNA antisense methods and chimeric dominant negative protein inhibitors.

Knockout Models

The most exhaustive studies with mammals have used embryonic stem (ES) cell technology to create knockout mice. With this technology, a selected gene is mutated in mouse ES cells in vitro. These mutated ES cells are then transferred back into preimplantation embryos, and mutant mice with the selected mutation are produced. Mice that carry this mutation are called "knockout" mice. If the gene of interest is normally expressed only in reproductive organs, then mice lacking this gene are expected to be viable without any defects outside the reproductive tract.

If a knockout mouse lacking a protein is fertile or subfertile, then that protein would be viewed as a less promising contraceptive target (i.e., humans in whom expression of that gene is blocked by drugs would also be fertile). However, if a knockout mouse lacking a protein is infertile, then that protein would be viewed as an excellent contraceptive target (i.e., blockade of this protein target in humans would demonstrate a contraceptive effect). Technology is now available to conditionally knockout expression of a gene in a specific tissue in adult mice. Use of this technology is ideal for the validation of contraceptive targets because the approach will more closely mimic the use of contraceptive targets by adults, and will also eliminate artifactual results due to developmental abnormalities.

In addition, if a gene is expressed specifically in the reproductive tract, there would be less of a chance for unwanted phenotypic effects elsewhere. A few examples of these mutations are described later in this chapter. Despite the progress in this area, funding is limited for reverse genetic screens based only on analysis of the reproductive tract-specific expression of a gene. The reason for this is that these gene-based screens are not viewed as hypothesis driven. However, these types of screens should be encouraged because extension of the screening database will provide more options for the identification of candidates with which to move forward for further validation.

RNA Interference

A new approach for studying the functions of specific genes is to reduce or eliminate gene expression through a process known as RNA interference (RNAi). RNAi is an innate cellular process that is initiated when a double-stranded RNA molecule enters the cell, causing the activation of proteins that destroy both the invading RNA and the endogenous single-stranded RNAs with identical sequences inside the cell. First identified in the nematode worm (*Caenorhabditis elegans*), this degradation pathway has since been found to operate in many organisms. The process most likely developed as a way to control pathogens and as a mechanism to control gene expression, but it has recently been harnessed by scientists as an efficient and powerful way to experimentally manipulate gene expression (reviewed by Hannon, 2002; Shuey et al., 2002). By designing appropriate double-stranded RNA molecules to match the sequence of a specific target mRNA, RNAi provides a relatively simple and fast way to block gene expression in experimental organisms as varied as plants, worms, flies, and mammals. For example, the RNAi approach has already been shown to be a useful technique for studying the functions of oocyte-specific genes and other RNA transcripts that play critical roles in oocyte maturation in mice (Stein et al., 2003; Svoboda et al., 2000). RNAi can also be used in high-throughput genetic screens to examine gene function on a whole-genome scale in organisms that range from worms to humans. Scientists are developing RNAi libraries that can be used to identify the relevant genes associated with a specific phenotype and also to subsequently confirm the functions of genes that have been identified.

Although application of the technology is still in its infancy, there is great optimism for the potential of this new tool. Nobel laureate Phillip Sharp, professor and director of the McGovern Institute for Brain Research at the Massachusetts Institute of Technology, calls RNAi the most important breakthrough in the past decade (Dutton and Perkel, 2003). However, cautious optimism is warranted, given the as yet unfulfilled expectations of past advances such as antisense RNA and ribozymes, other genetic tools used to inhibit gene expression. Furthermore, a recent study showed that small double-stranded RNA molecules can sometimes change the expression of nontarget genes, potentially confounding experimental results as well as therapeutic effects (Bridge et al., 2003; Jackson et al., 2003). Nonetheless, dozens of companies are banking on the promise of RNAi technology both as a research tool and for its potential in drug development (Dutton and Perkel, 2003). Several collaborations between biotechnology and pharmaceutical companies are under way to design gene- and transcript-specific inhibitors for gene function evaluation and target validation. Efforts are also under way to develop RNAi interventions to target viruses, inflammatory diseases, and metabolic diseases. Scientists have already shown the efficacy of RNAi in blocking viral replication, including that of HIV (Martinez et al., 2002), as well as disease states like hepatitis and cancer in experimental models (Agami, 2002; reviewed by Dutton and Perkel, 2003; Shuey et al., 2002). The first clinical trials are expected within the next few years.

Forward Genetic Screens

Another approach to the identification of important functional genes is the use of mutational screens. Known as forward genetics, this approach entails the induction of random mutations in an experimental cell or animal, identification of a relevant mutant phenotype, mapping and isolation of the gene that has been mutated, and finally, isolation and characterization of the protein encoded by the gene. Large-scale screens for mutations in the fruit fly (*Drosophila melanogaster*) recently led to the identification and classification of nearly 2,400 mutations that result in sterile males.[28] This collection of mutations has provided a wealth of material for defining the number and types of gene products that control the various aspects of male fertility, from germ cell formation and the development of sperm and eggs through fertilization and even into early embryonic

---

[28]Barbara T. Wakimoto, professor of biology, University of Washington, Seattle, in a presentation at the International Symposium on New Frontiers in Contraceptive Research, Washington, DC, July 15-16, 2003.

development. Because of the striking conservation of many molecular pathways used in animal cells of different species, the lessons learned from studies with *Drosophila* have enormous potential to enable discovery of the proteins required for sperm function in humans and thus may provide insight in the search for new contraceptives.

Studies that used a similar approach were recently undertaken with mice as well. For example, large-scale production of chemically induced mouse mutations has led to the identification of a number of mutations that affect fertility (Kile et al., 2003). In another study, a variety of mutations that affect essentially all stages of sperm and egg development have been identified, but more mutations were found to have an impact on male fertility than on female fertility.[29] On the basis of the results of these preliminary studies demonstrating the effectiveness of forward genetic screens for infertility mutant genes in mice, NIH has provided funding to conduct a large-scale project to isolate scores of infertility mutant genes that represent a substantial fraction of all genes required for mammalian fertility. The results will be made available to the scientific community for further study.

One limitation of forward genetics experiments is that they are very laborious and are thus quite expensive and time-consuming, even with current methods and technologies. In particular, the target of the gene in forward genetic mutagenesis screens is often difficult to identify. Hence, the development of alternative mutagenesis screens would be very helpful and should also be encouraged. One possible alternative is the transposon mutagenesis method developed by Largaespada and colleagues (Dupuy et al., 2002; Roberg-Perez et al., 2003). A transposon is a short sequence of DNA that can change location in the genome and normally contains genes that code for proteins that enable it to change location. By inserting a transposable element into the mouse germ line, scientists can induce the movement of the transposon into a new (random) location. If the transposon inserts into a location containing a gene, then the transposon should mutate this gene, thereby creating a novel mutation. Mice can be bred to homozygosity to evaluate the phenotypic effects of the mutation. By DNA sequence analysis, the new site of insertion of the transposon can be accurately determined. The Mouse Transposon Insertion Database[30] already has sequence data on 5,000 insertional mutations.

In a similar way, "genetrap" retroviral vectors have been invented to mutate genes in vitro in ES cells (Friedrich and Soriano, 1991; Hansen et

---

[29]John Schimenti, the Jackson Laboratory, in a presentation at the International Symposium on New Frontiers in Contraceptive Research, Washington, DC, July 15-16, 2003.
[30]See http://mouse.ccgb.umn.edu/transposon/ (accessed September 2003).

al., 2003). The site of the mutation (the trapped gene) can also be identified by DNA sequencing. The European ES Cell Consortium[31] has generated mutations in 11,000 genes in ES cells. These ES cells are publicly available.

PROMISING NEW TARGETS

There are many possible tissues and cells in the reproductive tract where inhibition or activation of gene product function could result in an infertility phenotype, and there are multiple options for either validation or rejection of target genes. Furthermore, after potential targets have been identified and validated, choosing the most promising targets for the next stages of drug discovery and development is enormously challenging. The drug development process is extremely costly and very risky, so wise selection of targets is essential to optimize the use of available funds and resources. A list of key criteria for target selection in contraception development is presented in Table 2.2.

The committee considered the following areas to be particularly promising for the discovery of new targets: the male spermatogenesis pathway, sperm maturation (both sperm and epididymal proteins), sperm capacitation, motility and chemotaxis in the female reproductive tract, proteins and molecules in the female reproductive system (vagina, cervix, uterus, and oviduct), sperm–egg interactions (both sperm and egg proteins and molecules), and maturation and ovulation of the egg (both somatic cell- and egg-specific proteins and molecules). The epithelium of the female reproductive tract is a prime target for contraceptive research, since sperm entry, transport, maturation, and sperm–egg interactions occur in the environment of this epithelium. The basic biologies of the epithelium of the vagina, the cervix, the endometrium, and the oviduct are fairly well understood with regard to the morphologic changes induced in these tissues by estrogen and progesterone. However, identification of targets for contraception by a genomics and subsequently proteomics approach is just beginning to be investigated. Several recent studies (Borthwick et al., 2003; Carson et al., 2002; Kao et al., 2002; Riesewijk et al., 2003) revealed potential targets in the human endometrium for inhibition of embryo implantation, including cell surface carbohydrate moieties, ion channels, essential element transporter proteins, and secretory proteins. Moreover, the role of the endometrial epithelium during sperm transport on its way to fertilize the egg is poorly understood and offers an important area of contraceptive target development. Likewise, identification of contraceptive targets in the epithelium of the vagina, cervix, and oviduct

---

[31]See http://genetrap.de (accessed September 2003).

TABLE 2.2 Defining the Key Criteria for Novel Contraceptive Target Selection

Criteria	Examples of Desirable Characteristics
Expression	Uniquely or selectively expressed in reproductive tract tissue or organs involved in reproduction
Function	Inhibiting function specifically and completely disrupts or alters a process unique to reproduction
Timing of action	Close to time of fertilization (e.g., postmeiotic events in gametogenesis)
Potential for reversible modulation by a drug	Druggable protein classes such as enzymes, membrane proteins, receptors, and ion channels and transporter proteins
Potential route of administration	Amenable to simple delivery systems ensuring ease of use and high rates of compliance
Potential for product manufacture	Inexpensive and easy to produce
Potential for noncontraceptive benefits	Dual protection against sexually transmitted infections and conception; protection against cancer or other diseases

is needed and constitutes an important area for further investigation. This approach may offer the advantage of localized delivery through the vagina to minimize potential systemic effects of compounds that may impair epithelial function.

It is clear from previous pharmaceutical development studies that specific types of proteins (e.g., receptors, ligands, enzymes, and ion channels or transporters; see Figure 2.1) would be excellent candidates as targets for drug development efforts in the near future (Drews, 2000). Thus, infertile knockout or knock-in mutant mouse models that lack or contain one of these types of proteins, respectively, would identify proteins with high priority as targets for drug development. In addition to the general mouse models described above, specific examples of these types of proteins are discussed in the next section. This list is not meant to be exhaustive, and the committee recognizes that new targets will emerge even before the publication of this document.

Sperm Chemotaxis

The sperm of marine invertebrates exhibits strong chemotaxis (attraction by chemicals) in response to a variety of signals. It has long been hypothesized that mammalian sperm may use similar mechanisms to find and fertilize an egg. The existence of sperm chemotaxis was first shown experimentally in rabbits by Dickmann (1963). Further experiments, also with rabbits, provided evidence that this phenomenon is triggered by the products of ovulation (Harper, 1973); and this has been confirmed by Fabro et al. (2002), who concluded that rabbit sperm are chemotactically attracted to follicular fluid. Earlier studies by the latter group showed that sperm accumulation in follicular fluid was the result of both sperm chemotaxis and chemokinesis, followed by hyperactivation of motility. They suggested that at least one chemotactic factor was a small (less than 10,000-dalton), nonhydrophobic molecule (Ralt et al., 1994) and that there was a sequential acquisition of a chemotactic response by human sperm (Cohen-Dayag et al., 1994).

A recent study indicates that human sperm also have the ability to detect and respond to chemotactic signals through a novel receptor called hOR17-4 (Spehr et al., 2003). This protein belongs to the olfactory receptor (OR) family, which includes 500 to 1,000 members that are expressed in the neural tissue of the nose. Despite the name, some ORs are also expressed in other tissues, but their role in these locations is unclear. About 50 ORs are known to be expressed in the testis, many predominantly or exclusively by cells involved in spermatogenesis. Although it has been known for some time that several OR proteins are present in sperm, their function has remained a mystery.

The recent study demonstrates that the newly identified sperm OR causes the sperm to navigate in a specific direction when it detects a concentration of specific laboratory chemicals, while other chemicals can act to block this specific movement (Spehr et al., 2003). However, the physiological chemical that attracts sperm in the female reproductive tract remains to be revealed. It is also not clear whether the physiological chemoattractant must necessarily be secreted by the egg or whether production by other cells or tissues in the female reproductive tract might suffice (or perhaps be even more efficient) in properly directing the sperm toward the egg in the oviduct. In any case, the data suggest that sperm chemotaxis may be a critical component of the fertilization process, and thus inhibition of the hOR17-4 signaling system could potentially block fertilization and serve as a novel contraceptive (Spehr et al., 2003). However, this hypothesis is controversial and needs further examination. If validated, the goal is to find a compound that, when placed in the female reproductive tract, would confuse the directional signals that sperm need to find and fertilize the egg. A better understanding of how the hOR17-4 signals the sperm to change direction or motility would be helpful in this regard, as the signaling pathways associated with OR proteins are generally quite complex (Babcock, 2003).

Sperm–Egg Interaction

Before fertilization, sperm must adhere to and fuse with the plasma membrane of the egg. Thus, molecules involved in these processes are candidate targets for new contraceptive development. With that goal in mind, a combination of experimental approaches has been used to determine the protein molecules on the surface of the sperm or egg required for adherence and fusion. Several proteins have been shown to play a role in adhesion, and these adhesion-mediating proteins likely function within the context of multimeric complexes at the cell surface (Evans and Florman, 2002; Primakoff and Myles, 2002; reviewed by Talbot et al., 2003). The molecular basis for the intercellular fusion, however, remains elusive. Some of the proteins involved in adherence were initially thought to play a role in fusion as well, but gene knockout studies have disproved that hypothesis.

Research on other proteins on the egg surface has pointed primarily in two directions.[32] Some proteins have a glycosylphosphatidylinositol (GPI) membrane anchor. GPI is a lipid that is attached to the protein and inserted into the lipid bilayer of the plasma membrane to anchor the protein on the surface of the cell. Proteins with this membrane anchor have been implicated in fusion because treatment of eggs with an enzyme that disrupts this anchor and releases these proteins from the surface results in eggs that do not fuse with sperm (Alfieri et al., 2003). Recent results show that female mice lacking the gene for an enzyme required to make the GPI membrane anchor (and that are therefore lacking GPI-anchored egg proteins on their surface) are infertile (Alfieri et al., 2003). These animals produce eggs that mature normally but are defective in sperm–egg fusion. Scientists are now searching for the particular GPI-anchored egg proteins that play a critical role in fusion and that could thus be suitable targets for contraceptives.

The second direction for research on proteins of the egg surface involves CD9, a member of the protein family called tetraspanins (because they cross the plasma membrane four times) that binds to integrins and facilitates cell proliferation, motility, and adhesion. Animals from which

---

[32]Diana Myles, Ph.D., University of California, Davis, in a presentation at the International Symposium on New Frontiers in Contraceptive Research, Washington, DC, July 15-16, 2003.

the gene for CD9 is deleted are infertile; their eggs cannot fuse with sperm. Ongoing efforts are aimed at determining what regions of the protein are directly involved in and essential for fusion and whether other proteins on the surface of the egg interact with CD9 to form a multiprotein structure or complex in the process of fusion (Zhu et al., 2002). Scientists are also searching for the protein on the surface of the sperm that interacts with CD9 on the egg.

Significant insight into the membrane fusion process has also come from studies of virus–cell fusion (Evans and Florman, 2002). Scientists have recently discovered the sites of fusion between HIV and other viruses in a host cell membrane. They have identified particular fusion proteins and have been gaining insights into how these proteins work. Importantly, precedent for therapeutic blocking of membrane fusion already exists in the literature. New drugs based on small peptides that can act as fusion inhibitors have been developed, and one of them, enfuvirtide (Kilby et al., 2002), was recently approved for use by the Food and Drug Administration. Although less is known about cell–cell fusion events, new insights are emerging from studies with sperm from sea urchins and abalone (Evans and Florman, 2002).

Proteins That Function in Gamete Metabolism and Maturation

Glyceraldehyde 3-phosphate dehydrogenase 2 (GAPDS or GAPD2) is an enzyme required for glycolysis (the breakdown of sugar to produce energy) that is expressed specifically in the testes of mice and humans (Welch et al., 2000). GAPDS is associated with the sperm tail. Because of the important role of GAPDS in glycolysis, male knockout mice lacking GAPDS are infertile. Sperm from these knockout mice have a motility defect (i.e., they do not have the normal "swimming" motion). This suggests that contraceptive drugs in the male or female reproductive tract that block GAPDS activity also would prevent the sperm from reaching an egg (Qu et al., 2003).

CKS2 is one of the mammalian cyclin-dependent kinase 1 binding protein homologues. Although this protein is expressed in multiple tissues, knockout mice lacking the gene for CKS2 have a normal phenotype, except that they are infertile (Spruck et al., 2003). The germ cells of both male and female mice fail to progress through the first meiotic metaphase, thereby preventing maturation of the germ cells and the eventual ability of gametes to undergo fertilization. Agents that target CKS2 or the other meiotic proteins that interact with CKS2 could be considered contraceptive drugs.

The egg protein known as zygote arrest 1 (ZAR1) is a novel oocyte-specific protein that was identified in sequence-based screens (Wu et al.,

2003a, b). The protein is highly conserved and specific to the oocytes of fish, frogs, rats, mice, and humans (Wu et al., 2003a, b). The *zar1* gene is a member of a class of genes called maternal effect genes, which are expressed in the maternal oocyte but which play a role after ovulation. The absence of the ZAR1 protein in the egg prevents the fusion of the male and female pronuclei, thereby arresting further development (Wu et al., 2003a). This results in infertility in females lacking the *zar1* gene. Blockade of the pathway in which the ZAR1 protein functions would be expected to cause a contraceptive effect.

Sperm Motility Proteins

Calcium ions play a major role in the regulation of sperm cell function. Recently, scientists discovered a novel family of proteins, known as CatSpers, that are uniquely expressed in male germ cells and that may form a multiprotein complex that regulates the influx of calcium into the sperm cell, thereby regulating motility (Lobley et al., 2003; Quill et al., 2001). These proteins are localized to the flagellum, and sperm motility is markedly decreased in mice that lack CatSper1. The male knockout mice are sterile because their sperm cannot fertilize intact eggs, but the animals are otherwise normal and healthy (Ren et al., 2001). Thus, molecules that target the CatSper proteins could potentially serve as an effective contraceptive.

Another protein, known as kinase anchoring protein (AKAP) 4 (Miki et al., 2002), is the major component of the sperm flagellum. *Akap4* is a male germ cell-specific gene that is transcribed only in the postmeiotic phase of spermatogenesis. AKAPs bind to the regulatory subunits of an enzyme called protein kinase A, as well as other proteins that control intercellular signal transduction pathways, such as kinases and phosphatases. Targeted deletion of the *akap4* gene in mice results in a male infertility phenotype (Miki et al., 2002). Sperm numbers were not reduced, but sperm failed to show progressive motility because of abnormal tail development. Consistent with the findings with the knockout mouse model, small peptides that block the protein kinase A regulatory subunit binding sites of AKAP cause sperm motility defects in bovine epididymal sperm (Vijayaraghavan et al., 1997), indicating that further efforts directed toward this protein as a potential contraceptive target should be pursued.

Hormone and Cytokine Signaling

The progesterone receptor mediates the genomic action of progesterone, a steroid hormone that is required for ovulation and preparation of the uterus for the process of implantation. The progesterone receptor gene gives rise to multiple proteins as a result of alternative transcription and translation start sites. The best-characterized progesterone receptor isoforms are the A and B forms. The A form is generally a repressor of transcription, whereas the B form is the longer protein and is a transcriptional activator. Female mice lacking progesterone receptors are infertile because of a defect in the process of ovulation as well as a uterine abnormality because of the inability to develop a receptive state and an associated inflammatory infiltration (Lydon et al., 1995). In the periovulatory period, progesterone receptors are induced in ovarian granulosa cells. Drugs that block periovulatory progesterone synthesis as well as progesterone receptor antagonists prevent ovulation (Shao et al., 2003). Collectively, these findings demonstrate that events that are initiated by progesterone and that act on the progesterone receptor are essential for the release of the oocyte from the mature follicle. Selective targeting experiments demonstrated that the progesterone receptor isoform required for ovulation is the A form (Mulac-Jericevic et al., 2000). The genes that are regulated by progesterone and that are essential for ovulation have yet to be elucidated, but analysis of differential gene expression through the study of transcript profiles of wild-type and progesterone receptor-deficient ovarian RNA suggests that degradative enzymes including cathepsin L and ADAMTS1 (a member of a family of proteins with a disintegrin and metalloprotease with thrombospondin type 1 repeat) are candidates for proteins that participate in the degradation of the follicle wall and thus release of the egg from the ovary (Richards et al., 2002; Robker et al., 2000). Understanding the gene and protein networks associated with progesterone action in the periovulatory period could yield new targets, including enzymes, for prevention of ovulation without disruption of ovarian endocrine activity.

A number of cytokines have also been identified as potential targets for development of anti-implantation strategies. For example, leukemia inhibitory factor (LIF) is essential for implantation in mice (Bhatt et al., 1991), and there is reason to believe that it plays a similar role in primates (Charnock-Jones et al., 1994; Chen et al., 1995; Cullinan et al., 1996; Vogiagis et al., 1996; Yue et al., 2000). Interleukin-11 (IL-11) is intimately involved in early decidualization in mice (Robb et al., 1998) and appears to play a similar role in humans (Dimitriadis et al., 2000, 2002). Work is under way to develop peptide inhibitors that block activation of the uterine LIF and IL-11 signaling pathways (Fairlie et al., 2002).

RECOMMENDATIONS

Major advances in identifying and verifying contraceptive targets in males and females have been made since publication of the 1996 Institute

of Medicine report. These targets are, in some cases, uniquely and exclusively involved in reproduction. The committee recognizes the existence
of several promising targets (i.e., proteins that have been shown to play
key roles in gamete maturation, function, or interactions) and strongly
recommends that these targets be pursued using high-throughput drug
discovery approaches (see Chapter 3). In addition, many more promising
targets can be expected from continued work in target discovery using a
variety of experimental approaches. Once these potential targets have
been identified, they will need to be validated in model organisms through
in depth phenotypic analysis using genomic and proteomic approaches.

**Recommendation 1: Identify and characterize all genes and proteins
uniquely or preferentially expressed in the testis, ovary, and reproductive tissues; and define the genetic and protein networks in cells
relevant to reproduction, including construction of a protein interaction map for the sperm and the egg.**

Emphasis should be placed on selective screening methods to identify classes of molecules that have been traditionally targeted by pharmaceutical compounds, including membrane proteins, enzymes, receptors,
and ion channels or transporter proteins. An achievable short-term goal
(less than 5 years) is the identification of all genes uniquely or preferentially expressed in all relevant reproductive cell and tissue types. This
could be accomplished in part through the provision of continued and
additional funding for a modest number of laboratories attempting to generate the reproductive transcriptome. However, to complete this task more
rapidly, the committee recommends that a broad group of reproductive
biologists, bioinformaticists, biochemists, and physiologists convene a
meeting with the sole purpose of verifying and annotating all gene
expression data obtained through genomic methods. The information
generated should then be stored in readily accessible World Wide Web-
based databases (e.g., the Mammalian Reproductive Genetics database,[33]
the Mouse Genome Informatics database,[34] or GermOnline[35]). Equally important, upkeep of the database will require vigilant review, annotation,
and standardization if it is to be a useful and valuable tool for the research
community (MacNeil, 2003).

In parallel with genomic approaches, the committee recognizes the
need, and unique opportunity, to apply proteomic methods to contraceptive research. One goal that is being pursued is the creation of sperm and

---

[33]See http://mrg.genetics.washington.edu/ (accessed September 2003).
[34]See http://www.informatics.jax.org/ (accessed September 2003).
[35]See http://www.germonline.unibas.ch/ (accessed January 2004).

egg proteome databases. However, this is a large undertaking that will require additional allocation of human resources and financial capital. Recognizing that genes and proteins do not act autonomously, the committee recommends that substantial new resources be devoted to identifying and constructing genetic and protein networks as well. This is a more long-term goal (greater than 5 years), but one that should be initiated immediately.

Genomic and proteomic approaches can also identify metabolic pathways and enzymes that are involved in the biosynthesis and catabolism of glycoproteins, glycolipids, and other lipids. Functional genomic approaches can reveal the importance of these pathways to reproductive processes. However, these techniques cannot establish the structures of unique carbohydrates on proteins and lipids or the content and organization of lipid domains within membranes. Consequently, different experimental methods are needed to characterize unique features of the glycomes and lipidomes of reproductive tract tissues and gametes.

Recommendation 2: Generate a lipidome and glycome of the reproductive tract tissues and mature gametes.

The glycomes and lipidomes of reproductive tract tissues and gametes have unique features not shared by other somatic tissues, and cell surface lipids and proteins represent logical targets for drugs, particularly small molecules that can interact with carbohydrate structures or insert in hydrophobic domains. Thus, the committee recommends that the investigation of the novel characteristics of the reproductive glycome and lipidome be pursued with the goal of identifying targets and small molecules that act to selectively disrupt membrane structure and function. The Consortium for Functional Glycomics, funded by the National Institute of General Medical Sciences, could provide useful research tools for an initiative in reproductive glycomics.

Recommendation 3: Validate existing and emerging contraceptive targets by using forward and reverse genetic approaches with model organisms.

Some of the identified targets described here will be validated or rejected during the normal progress of typical NIH-sponsored research programs. However, in some circumstances, study sections may not fund studies for the genetic validation of targets with unknown biochemical or molecular functions. To address this bottleneck, the committee recommends that a small consortium of investigators (public or private) be funded for the sole purpose of completing the genetic validation of all potential targets. To accomplish this goal most efficiently, newly established genetic models should be rapidly distributed to the community of scientists involved in reproductive biology research for prompt and comprehensive phenotypic analysis. Ideally, conditional gene knockout approaches should be used to reduce expression in specific adult tissues in order to replicate the use of contraceptives and to avoid artifacts due to developmental defects.

REFERENCES

Abe K, Ko MS, MacGregor GR. 1998. A systematic molecular genetic approach to study mammalian germline development. *Int J Dev Biol* 42(7 Spec No):1051–1065.

Agami R. 2002. RNAi and related mechanisms and their potential use for therapy. *Curr Opin Chem Biol* 6(6):829–834.

Akama TO, Nakagawa H, Sugihara K, Narisawa S, Ohyama C, Nishimura S, O'Brien DA, Moremen KW, Millan JL, Fukuda MN. 2002. Germ cell survival through carbohydrate-mediated interaction with Sertoli cells. *Science* 295(5552):124–127.

Alfieri JA, Martin AD, Takeda J, Kondoh G, Myles DG, Primakoff P. 2003. Infertility in female mice with an oocyte-specific knockout of GPI-anchored proteins. *J Cell Sci* 116(Pt 11):2149–2155.

Babcock DF. 2003. Development: smelling the roses? *Science* 299(5615):1993–1994.

Banerjee N, Zhang MQ. 2002. Functional genomics as applied to mapping transcription regulatory networks. *Curr Opin Microbiol* 5(3):313–317.

Bernstein GS. 1974. Physiological aspects of vaginal contraception. *Contraception* 9(4):333–345.

Bhatt H, Brunet LJ, Stewart CL. 1991. Uterine expression of leukemia inhibitory factor coincides with the onset of blastocyst implantation. *Proc Natl Acad Sci U S A* 88(24):11408–11412.

Boguski MS, McIntosh MW. 2003. Biomedical informatics for proteomics. *Nature* 422(6928):233–237.

Borthwick JM, Charnock-Jones DS, Tom BD, Hull ML, Teirney R, Phillips SC, Smith SK. 2003. Determination of the transcript profile of human endometrium. *Mol Hum Reprod* 9(1):19–33.

Brazhnik P, de la Fuente A, Mendes P. 2002. Gene networks: how to put the function in genomics. *Trends Biotechnol* 20(11):467–472.

Bridge AJ, Pebernard S, Ducraux A, Nicoulaz AL, Iggo R. 2003. Induction of an interferon response by RNAi vectors in mammalian cells. *Nat Genet* 34(3):263–264.

Burns KH, Owens GE, Ogbonna SC, Nilson JH, Matzuk MM. 2003. Expression profiling analyses of gonadotropin responses and tumor development in the absence of inhibins. *Endocrinology* 144(10):4492–4507.

Carson DD, Lagow E, Thathiah A, Al-Shami R, Farach-Carson MC, Vernon M, Yuan L, Fritz MA, Lessey B. 2002. Changes in gene expression during the early to mid-luteal (receptive phase) transition in human endometrium detected by high-density microarray screening. *Mol Hum Reprod* 8(9):871–879.

Charnock-Jones DS, Sharkey AM, Fenwick P, Smith SK. 1994. Leukaemia inhibitory factor mRNA concentration peaks in human endometrium at the time of implantation and the blastocyst contains mRNA for the receptor at this time. *J Reprod Fertil* 101(2):421–426.

Chen DB, Hilsenrath R, Yang ZM, Le SP, Kim SR, Chuong CJ, Poindexter AN III, Harper MJ. 1995. Leukaemia inhibitory factor in human endometrium during the menstrual cycle: cellular origin and action on production of glandular epithelial cell prostaglandin in vitro. *Hum Reprod* 10(4):911–918.

Chicurel ME, Dalma-Weiszhausz DD. 2002. Microarrays in pharmacogenomics: advances and future promise. *Pharmacogenomics* 3(5):589–601.

Chung S, Wang SP, Pan L, Mitchell G, Trasler J, Hermo L. 2001. Infertility and testicular defects in hormone-sensitive lipase-deficient mice. *Endocrinology* 142(10):4272–4281.

Cochran AG. 2000. Antagonists of protein-protein interactions. *Chem Biol* 7(4):R85–94.

Cohen-Dayag A, Ralt D, Tur-Kaspa I, Manor M, Makler A, Dor J, Mashiach S, Eisenbach M. 1994. Sequential acquisition of chemotactic responsiveness by human spermatozoa. *Biol Reprod* 50(4):786–790.

Cullinan EB, Abbondanzo SJ, Anderson PS, Pollard JW, Lessey BA, Stewart CL. 1996. Leukemia inhibitory factor (LIF) and LIF receptor expression in human endometrium suggests a potential autocrine/paracrine function in regulating embryo implantation. *Proc Natl Acad Sci U S A* 93(7):3115–3120.

Davis BK. 1976. Inhibitory effect of synthetic phospholipid vesicles containing cholesterol on the fertilizing ability of rabbit spermatozoa. *Proc Soc Exp Biol Med* 152(2):257–261.

Davis BK. 1980. Interaction of lipids with the plasma membrane of sperm cells, I: the antifertilization action of cholesterol. *Arch Androl* 5(3):249–254.

Davis BK. 1981. Timing of fertilization in mammals: sperm cholesterol/phospholipid ratio as a determinant of the capacitation interval. *Proc Natl Acad Sci U S A* 78(12):7560–7564.

Dickmann Z. 1963. Chemotaxis of rabbit spermatozoa. *J Exp Biol* 40:1–5.

Dimitriadis E, Salamonsen LA, Robb L. 2000. Expression of interleukin-11 during the human menstrual cycle: coincidence with stromal cell decidualization and relationship to leukaemia inhibitory factor and prolactin. *Mol Hum Reprod* 6(10):907–914.

Dimitriadis E, Robb L, Salamonsen LA. 2002. Interleukin 11 advances progesterone-induced decidualization of human endometrial stromal cells. *Mol Hum Reprod* 8(7):636–643.

Ding NZ, Ma XH, Diao HL, Xu LB, Yang ZM. 2003. Differential expression of peroxisome proliferator-activated receptor delta at implantation sites and in decidual cells of rat uterus. *Reproduction* 125(6):817–825.

Drews J. 2000. Drug discovery: a historical perspective. *Science* 287(5460):1960–1964.

Dupuy AJ, Clark K, Carlson CM, Fritz S, Davidson AE, Markley KM, Finley K, Fletcher CF, Ekker SC, Hackett PB, Horn S, Largaespada DA. 2002. Mammalian germ-line transgenesis by transposition. *Proc Natl Acad Sci U S A* 99(7):4495–4499.

Dutton G, Perkel JM. 2003. Shhh: silencing genes with RNA interference. *The Scientist* 17(7):42–44.

Evans JP, Florman HM. 2002. The state of the union: the cell biology of fertilization. *Nature Cell Biology* 4(S1):S57–S63 and *Nature Medicine* 8(S1)S57-S63.

Fabro G, Rovasio RA, Civalero S, Frenkel A, Caplan SR, Eisenbach M, Giojalas LC. 2002. Chemotaxis of capacitated rabbit spermatozoa to follicular fluid revealed by a novel directionality-based assay. *Biol Reprod* 67(5):1565–1571.

Fairlie WD, Uboldi AD, De Souza DP, Hemmings GJ, Nicola NA, Baca M. 2002. A fusion protein system for the recombinant production of short disulfide-containing peptides. *Protein Expr Purif* 26(1):171–178.

Fodor SP, Rava RP, Huang XC, Pease AC, Holmes CP, Adams CL. 1993. Multiplexed biochemical assays with biological chips. *Nature* 364(6437):555–556.

Friedrich G, Soriano P. 1991. Promoter traps in embryonic stem cells: a genetic screen to identify and mutate developmental genes in mice. *Genes Dev* 5(9):1513–1523.

Fujimoto H, Tadano-Aritomi K, Tokumasu A, Ito K, Hikita T, Suzuki K, Ishizuka I. 2000. Requirement of seminolipid in spermatogenesis revealed by UDP-galactose: ceramide galactosyltransferase-deficient mice. *J Biol Chem* 275(30):22623–22626.

Gahlay GK, Gupta SK. 2003. Glycosylation of zona pellucida glycoprotein-3 is required for inducing acrosomal exocytosis in the bonnet monkey. *Cell Mol Biol (Noisy-Le-Grand)* 49(3):389–397.

Giudice LC, Telles TL, Lobo S, Kao L. 2002. The molecular basis for implantation failure in endometriosis: on the road to discovery. *Ann N Y Acad Sci* 955:252–264; discussion 293–295, 396–406.

Habayeb OM, Bell SC, Konje JC. 2002. Endogenous cannabinoids: metabolism and their role in reproduction. *Life Sci* 70(17):1963–1977.

Halttunen M, Kamarainen M, Koistinen H. 2000. Glycodelin: a reproduction-related lipocalin. *Biochim Biophys Acta* 1482(1–2):149–156.

Hanash S. 2003. Disease proteomics. *Nature* 422(6928):226–232.

Hannon GJ. 2002. RNA interference. *Nature* 418(6894):244–251.

Hansen J, Floss T, Van Sloun P, Fuchtbauer EM, Vauti F, Arnold HH, Schnutgen F, Wurst W, von Melchner H, Ruiz P. 2003. A large-scale, gene-driven mutagenesis approach for the functional analysis of the mouse genome. *Proc Natl Acad Sci U S A* 100(17):9918–9922.

Harper MJ. 1973. Stimulation of sperm movement from the isthmus to the site of fertilization in the rabbit oviduct. *Biol Reprod* 8(3):362–368.

Harper MJ. 1989. Platelet-activating factor: a paracrine factor in preimplantation stages of reproduction? *Biol Reprod* 40(5):907–913.

Hasty J, McMillen D, Isaacs F, Collins JJ. 2001. Computational studies of gene regulatory networks: in numero molecular biology. *Nat Rev Genet* 2(4):268–279.

Honke K, Hirahara Y, Dupree J, Suzuki K, Popko B, Fukushima K, Fukushima J, Nagasawa T, Yoshida N, Wada Y, Taniguchi N. 2002. Paranodal junction formation and spermatogenesis require sulfoglycolipids. *Proc Natl Acad Sci U S A* 99(7):4227–4232.

Inaba K. 2003. Molecular architecture of the sperm flagella: molecules for motility and signaling. *Zoolog Sci* 20(9):1043–1056.

Institute of Medicine. 1996. *Contraceptive Research and Development: Looking to the Future*. Harrison PF, Rosenfield A, eds. Washington, DC: National Academy Press.

Institute of Medicine. 2003. *Large-Scale Biomedical Science: Exploring Strategies for Future Research*. Nass SJ, Stillman BW, eds. Washington, DC: The National Academies Press.

Ishii S, Shimizu T. 2000. Platelet-activating factor (PAF) receptor and genetically engineered PAF receptor mutant mice. *Prog Lipid Res* 39(1):41–82.

Ishii S, Nagase T, Shimizu T. 2002. Platelet-activating factor receptor. *Prostaglandins Other Lipid Mediat* 68-69:599–609.

Jackson AL, Bartz SR, Schelter J, Kobayashi SV, Burchard J, Mao M, Li B, Cavet G, Linsley PS. 2003. Expression profiling reveals off-target gene regulation by RNAi. *Nat Biotechnol* 21(6):635–637.

Jacobs KA, Collins-Racie LA, Colbert M, Duckett M, Golden-Fleet M, Kelleher K, Kriz R, LaVallie ER, Merberg D, Spaulding V, Stover J, Williamson MJ, McCoy JM. 1997. A genetic selection for isolating cDNAs encoding secreted proteins. *Gene* 198(1–2):289–296.

Jacobs KA, Collins-Racie LA, Colbert M, Duckett M, Evans C, Golden-Fleet M, Kelleher K, Kriz R, La Vallie ER, Merberg D, Spaulding V, Stover J, Williamson MJ, McCoy JM. 1999. A genetic selection for isolating cDNA clones that encode signal peptides. *Methods Enzymol* 303:468–479.

Kao LC, Tulac S, Lobo S, Imani B, Yang JP, Germeyer A, Osteen K, Taylor RN, Lessey BA, Giudice LC. 2002. Global gene profiling in human endometrium during the window of implantation. *Endocrinology* 143(6):2119–2138.

Kilby JM, Lalezari JP, Eron JJ, Carlson M, Cohen C, Arduino RC, Goodgame JC, Gallant JE, Volberding P, Murphy RL, Valentine F, Saag MS, Nelson EL, Sista PR, Dusek A. 2002. The safety, plasma pharmacokinetics, and antiviral activity of subcutaneous enfuvirtide (T-20), a peptide inhibitor of gp41-mediated virus fusion, in HIV-infected adults. *AIDS Res Hum Retrovir* 18(10):685–693.

Kile BT, Hentges KE, Clark AT, Nakamura H, Salinger AP, Liu B, Box N, Stockton DW, Johnson RL, Behringer RR, Bradley A, Justice MJ. 2003. Functional genetic analysis of mouse chromosome 11. *Nature* 425(6953):81–86.

Kleene KC. 2001. A possible meiotic function of the peculiar patterns of gene expression in mammalian spermatogenic cells. *Mech Dev* 106(1–2):3–23.

Ko MS, Kitchen JR, Wang X, Threat TA, Wang X, Hasegawa A, Sun T, Grahovac MJ, Kargul GJ, Lim MK, Cui Y, Sano Y, Tanaka T, Liang Y, Mason S, Paonessa PD, Sauls AD, DePalma GE, Sharara R, Rowe LB, Eppig J, Morrell C, Doi H. 2000. Large-scale cDNA analysis reveals phased gene expression patterns during preimplantation mouse development. *Development* 127(8):1737–1749.

Koyanagi R, Honegger TG. 2003. Molecular cloning and sequence analysis of an ascidian egg beta-N-acetylhexosaminidase with a potential role in fertilization. *Dev Growth Differ* 45(3):209–218.

Leo CP, Pisarska MD, Hsueh AJ. 2001. DNA array analysis of changes in preovulatory gene expression in the rat ovary. *Biol Reprod* 65(1):269–276.

Li DK, Liu L, Odouli R. 2003. Exposure to non-steroidal anti-inflammatory drugs during pregnancy and risk of miscarriage: population based cohort study. *BMJ* 327(7411):368.

Lim H, Dey SK. 2000. PPAR delta functions as a prostacyclin receptor in blastocyst implantation. *Trends Endocrinol Metab* 11(4):137–142.

Lim H, Dey SK. 2002. A novel pathway of prostacyclin signaling–hanging out with nuclear receptors. *Endocrinology* 143(9):3207–3210.

Lim H, Paria BC, Das SK, Dinchuk JE, Langenbach R, Trzaskos JM, Dey SK. 1997. Multiple female reproductive failures in cyclooxygenase 2-deficient mice. *Cell* 91(2):197–208.

Lobley A, Pierron V, Reynolds L, Allen L, Michalovich D. 2003. Identification of human and mouse CatSper3 and CatSper4 genes: characterisation of a common interaction domain and evidence for expression in testis. *Reprod Biol Endocrinol* 1(1):53.

Logan JE, Roudebush WE. 2000. Platelet-activating factor increases intracellular calcium levels in preimplantation stage embryos. *Early Pregnancy* 4(1):30–38.

Lydon JP, DeMayo FJ, Funk CR, Mani SK, Hughes AR, Montgomery CA Jr, Shyamala G, Conneely OM, O'Malley BW. 1995. Mice lacking progesterone receptor exhibit pleiotropic reproductive abnormalities. *Genes Dev* 9(18):2266–2278.

Maccarrone M, Bisogno T, Valensise H, Lazzarin N, Fezza F, Manna C, Di Marzo V, Finazzi-Agro A. 2002. Low fatty acid amide hydrolase and high anandamide levels are associated with failure to achieve an ongoing pregnancy after IVF and embryo transfer. *Mol Hum Reprod* 8(2):188–195.

MacNeil JS. 2003. Molecular databases grow, and grow, . . . and grow. *The Scientist* 17(15):40–44.

Margolin J. 2001. From comparative and functional genomics to practical decisions in the clinic: a view from the trenches. *Genome Res* 11(6):923–925.

Marions L, Viski S, Danielsson KG, Resch BA, Swahn ML, Bygdeman M, Kovacs L. 1999. Contraceptive efficacy of daily administration of 0.5 mg mifepristone. *Hum Reprod* 14(11):2788–2790.

Martinez MA, Clotet B, Este JA. 2002. RNA interference of HIV replication. *Trends Immunol* 23(12):559–561.

Matsumoto H, Ma W, Smalley W, Trzaskos J, Breyer RM, Dey SK. 2001. Diversification of cyclooxygenase-2-derived prostaglandins in ovulation and implantation. *Biol Reprod* 64(5):1557–1565.

Matzuk MM, Lamb DJ. 2002. Genetic dissection of mammalian fertility pathways. *Nature Cell Biology* 4(S1):S41–S49 and *Nature Medicine* 8(S1)S41–S49.

McCarrey JR, O'Brien DA, Skinner MK. 1999. Construction and preliminary characterization of a series of mouse and rat testis cDNA libraries. *J Androl* 20(5):635–639.

McCauley TC, Kurth BE, Norton EJ, Klotz KL, Westbrook VA, Rao AJ, Herr JC, Diekman AB. 2002. Analysis of a human sperm CD52 glycoform in primates: identification of an animal model for immunocontraceptive vaccine development. *Biol Reprod* 66(6):1681–1688.

McLean DJ, Friel PJ, Pouchnik D, Griswold MD. 2002. Oligonucleotide microarray analysis of gene expression in follicle-stimulating hormone-treated rat Sertoli cells. *Mol Endocrinol* 16(12):2780–2792.

Miki K, Willis WD, Brown PR, Goulding EH, Fulcher KD, Eddy EM. 2002. Targeted disruption of the *akap4* gene causes defects in sperm flagellum and motility. *Dev Biol* 248(2):331–342.

Mulac-Jericevic B, Mullinax RA, DeMayo FJ, Lydon JP, Conneely OM. 2000. Subgroup of reproductive functions of progesterone mediated by progesterone receptor-B isoform. *Science* 289(5485):1751–1754.

Muramatsu T. 2002. Development: carbohydrate recognition in spermatogenesis. *Science* 295(5552):53–54.

Nayak S, Galili N, Buck CA. 1998. Immunohistochemical analysis of the expression of two serine-threonine kinases in the maturing mouse testis. *Mech Dev* 74(1–2):171–174.

Neilson L, Andalibi A, Kang D, Coutifaris C, Strauss JF III, Stanton JA, Green DP. 2000. Molecular phenotype of the human oocyte by PCR-SAGE. *Genomics* 63(1):13–24.

Osuga J, Ishibashi S, Oka T, Yagyu H, Tozawa R, Fujimoto A, Shionoiri F, Yahagi N, Kraemer FB, Tsutsumi O, Yamada N. 2000. Targeted disruption of hormone-sensitive lipase results in male sterility and adipocyte hypertrophy, but not in obesity. *Proc Natl Acad Sci U S A* 97(2):787–792.

Paria BC, Dey SK. 2000. Ligand-receptor signaling with endocannabinoids in preimplantation embryo development and implantation. *Chem Phys Lipids* 108(1–2):211–220.

Paria BC, Wang H, Dey SK. 2002. Endocannabinoid signaling in synchronizing embryo development and uterine receptivity for implantation. *Chem Phys Lipids* 121(1–2):201–210.

Pawson T, Nash P. 2003. Assembly of cell regulatory systems through protein interaction domains. *Science* 300(5618):445–452.

Penttinen J, Pujianto DA, Sipila P, Huhtaniemi I, Poutanen M. 2003. Discovery in silico, and characterization in vitro of novel genes exclusively expressed in the mouse epididymis. *Mol Endocrinol* 17(11):2138–2151.

Phizicky E, Bastiaens PI, Zhu H, Snyder M, Fields S. 2003. Protein analysis on a proteomic scale. *Nature* 422(6928):208–215.

Primakoff P, Myles DG. 2002. Penetration, adhesion, and fusion in mammalian sperm–egg interaction. *Science* 296(5576):2183–2185.

Qu WD, Miki K, O'Brien DA. 2003. *Tyrosine Phosphorylation of High Molecular Weight Proteins Is Impaired in Glyceraldehyde 3-Phosphate Dehydrogenase-S (GAPDS) Knockout Mice.* Presented at the XVII Testis Workshop: Functional genomics of male reproduction. Phoenix, AZ, March 26–29.

Quill TA, Ren D, Clapham DE, Garbers DL. 2001. A voltage-gated ion channel expressed specifically in spermatozoa. *Proc Natl Acad Sci U S A* 98(22):12527–12531.

Rajkovic A, Yan M S C, Klysik M, Matzuk M. 2001. Discovery of germ cell–specific transcripts by expressed sequence tag database analysis. *Fertil Steril* 76(3):550–554.

Ralt D, Manor M, Cohen-Dayag A, Tur-Kaspa I, Ben-Shlomo I, Makler A, Yuli I, Dor J, Blumberg S, Mashiach S. 1994. Chemotaxis and chemokinesis of human spermatozoa to follicular factors. *Biol Reprod* 50(4):774–785.

Rankin TL, Tong ZB, Castle PE, Lee E, Gore-Langton R, Nelson LM, Dean J. 1998. Human ZP3 restores fertility in Zp3 null mice without affecting order-specific sperm binding. *Development* (13):2415–2424.

Ren D, Navarro B, Perez G, Jackson AC, Hsu S, Shi Q, Tilly JL, Clapham DE. 2001. A sperm ion channel required for sperm motility and male fertility. *Nature* 413(6856):603–609.

Richards JS, Russell DL, Ochsner S, Hsieh M, Doyle KH, Falender AE, Lo YK, Sharma SC. 2002. Novel signaling pathways that control ovarian follicular development, ovulation, and luteinization. *Recent Prog Horm Res* 57:195–220.

Riesewijk A, Martin J, van Os R, Horcajadas JA, Polman J, Pellicer A, Mosselman S, Simon C. 2003. Gene expression profiling of human endometrial receptivity on days LH+2 versus LH+7 by microarray technology. *Mol Hum Reprod* 9(5):253–264.

Robb L, Li R, Hartley L, Nandurkar HH, Koentgen F, Begley CG. 1998 . Infertility in female mice lacking the receptor for interleukin 11 is due to a defective uterine response to implantation. *Nat Med* 4(3):303–308.

Roberg-Perez K, Carlson CM, Largaespada DA. 2003. MTID: a database of Sleeping Beauty transposon insertions in mice. *Nucleic Acids Res* 31(1):78–81.

Robker RL, Russell DL, Espey LL, Lydon JP, O'Malley BW, Richards JS. 2000. Progesterone-regulated genes in the ovulation process: ADAMTS-1 and cathepsin L proteases. *Proc Natl Acad Sci U S A* 97(9):4689–4694.

Rodemer C, Thai TP, Brugger B, Kaercher T, Werner H, Nave KA, Wieland F, Gorgas K, Just WW. 2003. Inactivation of ether lipid biosynthesis causes male infertility, defects in eye development and optic nerve hypoplasia in mice. *Hum Mol Genet* 12(15):1881–1895.

Sali A, Glaeser R, Earnest T, Baumeister W. 2003. From words to literature in structural proteomics. *Nature* 422(6928):216–225.

Schena M, Shalon D, Heller R, Chai A, Brown PO, Davis RW. 1996. Parallel human genome analysis: microarray-based expression monitoring of 1000 genes. *Proc Natl Acad Sci U S A* 93(20):10614–10619.

Schlecht U, Primig M. 2003. Mining meiosis and gametogenesis with DNA microarrays. *Reproduction* 125(4):447–456.

Schuel H, Burkman LJ, Lippes J, Crickard K, Forester E, Piomelli D, Giuffrida A. 2002. N-Acylethanolamines in human reproductive fluids. *Chem Phys Lipids* 121(1–2):211–227.

Schultz N, Hamra FK, Garbers DL. 2003. A multitude of genes expressed solely in meiotic or postmeiotic spermatogenic cells offers a myriad of contraceptive targets. *Proc Natl Acad Sci U S A* 100(21):12201–12206.

Service RF. 2003. American Chemical Society meeting: arraymaker speeds analyses by months. *Science* 302(5642):47.

Shao R, Markstrom E, Friberg PA, Johansson M, Billig H. 2003. Expression of progesterone receptor (PR) A and B isoforms in mouse granulosa cells: stage-dependent PR-mediated regulation of apoptosis and cell proliferation. *Biol Reprod* 68(3):914–921.

Shinkai Y, Satoh H, Takeda N, Fukuda M, Chiba E, Kato T, Kuramochi T, Araki Y. 2002. A testicular germ cell–associated serine-threonine kinase, MAK, is dispensable for sperm formation. *Mol Cell Biol* 22(10):3276–3280.

Shuey DJ, McCallus DE, Giordano T. 2002. RNAi: gene-silencing in therapeutic intervention. *Drug Discov Today* 7(20):1040–1046.

Snyder M, Gerstein M. 2003. Genomics: defining genes in the genomics era. *Science* 300(5617):258–260.

Spehr M, Gisselmann G, Poplawski A, Riffell JA, Wetzel CH, Zimmer RK, Hatt H. 2003. Identification of a testicular odorant receptor mediating human sperm chemotaxis. *Science* 299(5615):2054–2058.

Spruck CH, de Miguel MP, Smith AP, Ryan A, Stein P, Schultz RM, Lincoln AJ, Donovan PJ, Reed SI. 2003. Requirement of CKS2 for the first metaphase/anaphase transition of mammalian meiosis. *Science* 300(5619):647–650.

Srivastav A. 2000. Maturation-dependent glycoproteins containing both N- and O-linked oligosaccharides in epididymal sperm plasma membrane of rhesus monkeys (*Macaca mulatta*). *J Reprod Fertil* 119(2):241–252.

Stein P, Svoboda P, Schultz RM. 2003. Transgenic RNAi in mouse oocytes: a simple and fast approach to study gene function. *Dev Biol* 256(1):187–193.

Suzumori N, Burns KH, Yan W, Matzuk MM. 2003. RFPL4 interacts with oocyte proteins of the ubiquitin-proteasome degradation pathway. *Proc Natl Acad Sci U S A* 100(2):550–555.

Svoboda P, Stein P, Hayashi H, Schultz RM. 2000. Selective reduction of dormant maternal mRNAs in mouse oocytes by RNA interference. *Development* 127(19):4147–4156.

Taft RA, Denegre JM, Pendola FL, Eppig JJ. 2002. Identification of genes encoding mouse oocyte secretory and transmembrane proteins by a signal sequence trap. *Biol Reprod* 67(3):953–960.

Takamiya K, Yamamoto A, Furukawa K, Zhao J, Fukumoto S, Yamashiro S, Okada M, Haraguchi M, Shin M, Kishikawa M, Shiku H, Aizawa S, Furukawa K. 1998. Complex gangliosides are essential in spermatogenesis of mice: possible roles in the transport of testosterone. *Proc Natl Acad Sci U S A* 95(21):12147–12152.

Talbot P, Shur BD, Myles DG. 2003. Cell adhesion and fertilization: steps in oocyte transport, sperm-zona pellucida interactions, and sperm–egg fusion. *Biol Reprod* 68(1):1–9.

Tanaka H, Yoshimura Y, Nozaki M, Yomogida K, Tsuchida J, Tosaka Y, Habu T, Nakanishi T, Okada M, Nojima H, Nishimune Y. 1999. Identification and characterization of a haploid germ cell–specific nuclear protein kinase (Haspin) in spermatid nuclei and its effects on somatic cells. *J Biol Chem* 274(24):17049–17057.

Toledo AA, Mitchell-Leef D, Elsner CW, Slayden SM, Roudebush WE. 2003. Fertilization potential of human sperm is correlated with endogenous platelet-activating factor content. *J Assist Reprod Genet* 20(5):192–195.

Travis AJ, Kopf GS. 2002. The role of cholesterol efflux in regulating the fertilization potential of mammalian spermatozoa. *J Clin Invest* 110:731–736.

Trigatti B, Rayburn H, Vinals M, Braun A, Miettinen H, Penman M, Hertz M, Schrenzel M, Amigo L, Rigotti A, Krieger M. 1999. Influence of the high density lipoprotein receptor SR-BI on reproductive and cardiovascular pathophysiology. *Proc Natl Acad Sci U S A* 96(16):9322–9327.

Tsuji Y, Fukuda H, Iuchi A, Ishizuka I, Isojima S. 1992. Sperm immobilizing antibodies react to the 3-O-sulfated galactose residue of seminolipid on human sperm. *J Reprod Immunol* 22(3):225–236.

Tyers M, Mann M. 2003. From genomics to proteomics. *Nature* 422(6928):193–197.

Van den Nieuwenhof IM, Koistinen H, Easton RL, Koistinen R, Kamarainen M, Morris HR, Van Die I, Seppala M, Dell A, Van den Eijnden DH. 2000. Recombinant glycodelin carrying the same type of glycan structures as contraceptive glycodelin-A can be produced in human kidney 293 cells but not in Chinese hamster ovary cells. *Eur J Biochem* 267(15):4753–4762.

van der Spoel AC, Jeyakumar M, Butters TD, Charlton HM, Moore HD, Dwek RA, Platt FM. 2002. Reversible infertility in male mice after oral administration of alkylated imino sugars: a nonhormonal approach to male contraception. *Proc Natl Acad Sci U S A* 99(26):17173–17178.

van Someren EP, Wessels LF, Backer E, Reinders MJ. 2002. Genetic network modeling. *Pharmacogenomics* 3(4):507–525.

Vidal M. 2001. A biological atlas of functional maps. *Cell* 104(3):333–339.

Vijayaraghavan S, Olson GE, NagDas S, Winfrey VP, Carr DW. 1997. Subcellular localization of the regulatory subunits of cyclic adenosine 3',5'-monophosphate-dependent protein kinase in bovine spermatozoa. *Biol Reprod* 57(6):1517–1523.

Vo LH, Yen TY, Macher BA, Hedrick JL. 2003. Identification of the ZPC oligosaccharide ligand involved in sperm binding and the glycan structures of *Xenopus laevis* vitelline envelope glycoproteins. *Biol Reprod* 69(6):1822–1830.

Vogiagis D, Marsh MM, Fry RC, Salamonsen LA. 1996. Leukaemia inhibitory factor in human endometrium throughout the menstrual cycle. *J Endocrinol* 148(1):95–102.

Wang PJ, McCarrey JR, Yang F, Page DC. 2001. An abundance of X-linked genes expressed in spermatogonia. *Nat Genet* 27(4):422–426.

Wassarman PM. 2002. Sperm receptors and fertilization in mammals. *Mt Sinai J Med* 69(3):148–155.

Welch JE, Brown PL, O'Brien DA, Magyar PL, Bunch DO, Mori C, Eddy EM. 2000. Human glyceraldehyde 3-phosphate dehydrogenase-2 gene is expressed specifically in spermatogenic cells. *J Androl* 21(2):328–338.

Wilson JF. 2003. Long-suffering lipids gain respect: technical advances and enhanced understanding of lipid biology fuel a trend toward lipidomics. *The Scientist* 17(5):34–36.

Wu X, Viveiros MM, Eppig JJ, Bai Y, Fitzpatrick SL, Matzuk MM. 2003a. Zygote arrest 1 (Zar1) is a novel maternal-effect gene critical for the oocyte-to-embryo transition. *Nat Genet* 33(2):187–191.

Wu X, Wang P, Brown CA, Zilinski CA, Matzuk MM. 2003b. Zygote arrest 1 (Zar1) is an evolutionarily conserved gene expressed in vertebrate ovaries. *Biol Reprod* 69(3):861–867.

Yue ZP, Yang ZM, Wei P, Li SJ, Wang HB, Tan JH, Harper MJ. 2000. Leukemia inhibitory factor, leukemia inhibitory factor receptor, and glycoprotein 130 in rhesus monkey uterus during menstrual cycle and early pregnancy. *Biol Reprod* 63(2):508–512.

Zhu GZ, Miller BJ, Boucheix C, Rubinstein E, Liu CC, Hynes RO, Myles DG, Primakoff P. 2002. Residues SFQ (173-175) in the large extracellular loop of CD9 are required for gamete fusion. *Development* 129(8):1995–2002.

3

Product Identification and Development

Men and women need new options for contraception. The products marketed at present are limited in their modes of action, are not 100% effective even if used correctly, can be difficult to use correctly and consistently, in many cases produce unwanted side effects, and do not provide the wide range of choices desired by both women and men at different stages of their lives. The 1996 report of the Institute of Medicine on contraceptive development recommended that new approaches to both female- and male-based contraceptives be developed by capitalizing on many of the emerging scientific technologies as well as discoveries being made in university-based laboratories. However, the report did not address in detail how such discoveries could be translated into products, since the public sector is clearly limited in its ability to develop and bring such products to market.

A key component in the development and commercialization of new generations of contraceptives is identification of both new targets and molecular entities to modulate those targets. Moreover, the ability to validate those targets, identify promising drug candidates, and provide the vast amount of preclinical and clinical data necessary to meet the regulatory requirements needed before marketing requires a complex and costly organizational infrastructure. Given the documented need for low-cost contraceptives for much of the world's population, the development and testing of such contraceptives are not likely to be achieved by government or public-sector programs alone and will require substantial participation of the pharmaceutical industry. A conundrum lies in the fact that the present lack of financial incentives for the pharmaceutical industry to develop such products remains an important limitation to interest by the industry.

The committee considered several different issues related to this problem, which are listed below, and addresses each of these issues in this chapter:

1. How might the discovery of compounds that modulate existing and emerging targets be accelerated or made more effective?

2. How might the movement of novel lead compounds through development and into clinical trials be enhanced and accelerated?

3. How can current delivery systems be maximally used and how can new delivery systems be developed for new contraceptives?

4. How can the pharmaceutical and biotechnology industries be more effectively engaged in all aspects of target selection, compound identification, development, and clinical investigation?

MOVING FROM TARGET SELECTION TO PRODUCT DEVELOPMENT

After potential new targets for contraceptives have been identified, scientists still face enormous challenges in identifying and moving compounds forward to the clinic and subsequent widespread therapeutic use. To begin with, a target must be validated. That is, it must be convincingly demonstrated that changing the expression or activity of the target will lead to the desired outcome. Companies are unlikely to invest in the development of drugs directed at novel targets unless there is strong evidence for the likelihood that pharmaceutical manipulation of that target will be successful and lead to the expected clinical outcome.[1]

The U.S. pharmaceutical industry's traditional "success rate"—the fraction of Investigational New Drugs (INDs) that proceed to New Drug Applications (NDAs) through the Food and Drug Administration (FDA)—is about 1 in 5, or 20 percent. However, there is considerable variation within that average, depending on whether the drug was acquired from outside the United States (Dimasi, 2001). If it originated and was first tested elsewhere (that is, it was essentially prescreened), the average success rate with regard to approval by the FDA is 1 in 3; if the product originated in the United States but was first tested abroad, the success rate is 1 in 6; and if it both originated and was first tested in the United

---

[1]Charles Grudzinskas, Ph.D., drug development consultant, and adjunct professor, Georgetown University, in a presentation at the International Symposium on New Frontiers in Contraceptive Research, Washington, DC, July 15-16, 2003.

States, the rate is 1 in 12. Clearly, these rates can influence companies' strategies for developing new pharmaceuticals. Success rates also vary by therapeutic area (Dimasi, 2001). Although contraceptives were not examined as a specific category in this analysis, one could predict that the success rates for new contraceptive drugs might be relatively low, given that they must be inordinately safe if they are to be used by healthy individuals for long periods of time.

Drug development efforts can fail for a variety of reasons. On average, only about 20 percent of compounds for which an IND is filed successfully proceed to new drug approval (Figure 3.1). For roughly 35 to 40 percent of test compounds, development efforts fail because of insufficient efficacy. Economics plays a role about 30 to 35 percent of the time, as potential partners believe that they cannot successfully commercialize the drug. Lastly, safety concerns lead to the termination of drug development efforts about 20 percent of the time (Dimasi, 2001).

In any case, the drug development process is lengthy and expensive. The time needed to obtain FDA approval once testing with humans has begun ranges from 7 to 10 years, on average. In the United States, the

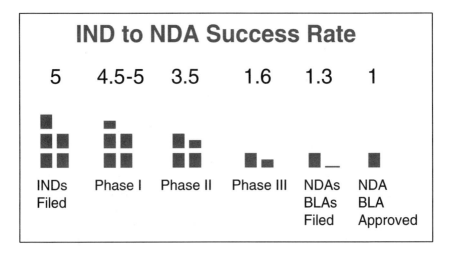

FIGURE 3.1 Success rate in moving from an investigational new drug (IND) application to a new drug application (NDA) or biologics license application (BLA).
SOURCE: Charles Grudzinskas, drug development consultant and adjunct professor, Georgetown University, in a presentation at the International Symposium on New Frontiers in Contraceptive Research, Washington, DC, July 15-16, 2003.

approval of a new contraceptive for women usually requires the submission of data for a total of 10,000 cycles of use, which should include data for 200 women who have completed 1 full year of therapy. For long-term delivery systems, the duration of follow-up depends on the duration of action of that system (e.g., 3 to 5 years for an implant or an intrauterine system). European regulations require data on a total of 20,000 cycles of use, which should include data for 400 women who have completed 1 full year of therapy. In contrast, no such guidelines exist for male contraceptives. The cost required to develop a successful compound is generally about $100 million to $150 million, but the total cost of new drug development can approach $800 million (taking into account the time and money invested in failures in the development process). For that reason, companies hope that candidate drugs destined for failure will fail early in the process (i.e., before clinical development) and thus limit their investment. The goal is to conduct critical experiments early to identify as soon as possible projects that would otherwise fail later in the clinical development process.

In addition to evidence of target validation, a wide variety of issues must be considered before a commitment is made to begin commercial drug development (Box 3.1). One important issue is determination of how the intended new drug's product profile will distinguish it from products already on the market. Important advantages could be improved safety, effectiveness, tolerability, compliance, continuation rate, and access. Pharmacogenetics must also be considered as a way to improve both safety and efficacy. Pharmacogenetics refers to the natural genetic variations in humans that can determine who will have an efficacious response and who will have a deleterious response to a particular drug. A prismatic example of the impact of ethnicity or genetics on contraceptive development is the difference in the level of suppression of spermatogenesis caused by exogenous testosterone, which is greater in Chinese men than Caucasian men (reviewed by Waites, 2003). The cause for this difference by ethnicity is not yet known.

In the past, pharmacogenetic variation was difficult or impossible to predict, but new tools and diagnostic methods are emerging to identify which individuals are most likely to experience a positive or a negative effect from a drug. Furthermore, the FDA recently issued the first guidelines that encourage drug and biologic developers to conduct pharmacogenetic tests during drug development and clarify how FDA will evaluate the resulting data (Food and Drug Administration, 2003).

BOX 3.1
Examples of Key Questions to Address in Deciding Whether to Pursue the Development of a Novel Drug

- Who should take this drug?
- What dose is needed?
- How often and how long will it need to be taken?
- What happens if a dose is missed?
- What kinds of side effects can be expected? Are they reversible?
- Are there any patients who should not take the drug?
- Are there any other drugs that are incompatible with this one?
- Will some individuals metabolize it differently so that only they will have drug–drug interactions?
- Is the drug highly protein bound?
- Will other drugs compete with and increase or decrease this drug's levels in blood, or conversely, will this drug compete and raise or lower the blood levels of another drug that the patient is taking?
- What happens when the patient suddenly stops taking the drug (or misses a few doses)? Is there a rebound?
- Is the drug addictive?
- Will dose need to be adjusted in people who have renal or hepatic impairment?
- Will food have any effect on the levels of the drug in blood?
- If the dose of the drug is doubled, will the levels in blood also double? (and what if the dose is tripled or increased only by 50 percent—or less?)
- What will be the drug's shelf life?

SOURCE: Charles Grudzinskas, drug development consultant and adjunct professor, Georgetown University, in a presentation at the International Symposium on New Frontiers in Contraceptive Research, Washington, DC, July 15-16, 2003.

EXAMPLES OF TECHNOLOGICAL ADVANCES IN DRUG DEVELOPMENT

Advances in Methods for Production of Pharmaceutical Proteins

Biotechnology and pharmaceutical companies are testing a number of human antibodies and other proteins as potential therapeutic compounds. Proteins and peptides are excellent therapeutic agents, as exemplified by the widespread use of natural substances such as insulin for diabetes, growth hormone for growth deficiencies, and most recently, parathyroid hormone for osteoporosis. Erythropoietin has achieved high regard for its utility in the treatment of anemia and as an adjunct to cancer chemotherapy, and activated protein C has been used to treat sepsis. Peptide agonists of the gonadotropin-releasing hormone receptor have been useful in treating hormone dependent proliferative diseases such as endometriosis, prostate cancer, and breast cancer. Human antibodies have been shown to have therapeutic efficacy and are currently marketed for several indications, such as Crohn's disease and rheumatoid arthritis (infliximab), psoriasis (efalizumab), non-Hodgkin's lymphoma (rituximab), and breast cancer (trastuzumab). They have also been used as adjunctive therapy with percutaneous angioplasty (abciximab). The most common antibody therapeutics are monoclonal antibodies, which are uniform antibodies that recognize only one specific target. Although most antibody-based therapies have been directed toward cancer and autoimmune–inflammation conditions, many are also under development for the treatment of infectious diseases and Alzheimer's disease. Furthermore, antibodies have the potential to prevent the transmission of sexually transmitted infections (STIs) (Veazey et al., 2003; Zeitlin et al., 2002). Because monoclonal antibodies have been established as viable, clinically useful modalities, there is a strong potential for the development of antibodies as contraceptive agents as well.[2]

Advantages of Antibodies

Monoclonal antibodies have two features that are particularly desirable for drug application: persistence and the ability to agglutinate (clump) cells. Monoclonal antibodies persist because they have half-lives of about 20 days, which is longer than those of other classes of therapeutic molecules (Table 3.1). A long half-life could reduce the rate of failure of a contraceptive due to imperfect use. That is, if one fails to use it on a given day, there will still be adequate protection from the previous day's dose. The agglutination ability of monoclonal antibodies allow them to agglutinate sperm, which can block fertilization by preventing the sperm from migrating through cervical mucus (Castle et al., 1997). In fact, the presence of agglutinating antibodies is one of the diagnostics for a woman who is infertile because of immunity.

---

[2]Kevin Whaley, Ph.D., Johns Hopkins University, ReProtect, Inc., Epicyte Pharmaceutical, Inc., Mapp Biopharmaceutical, Inc., in a presentation at the International Symposium on New Frontiers in Contraceptive Research, Washington, DC, July 15-16, 2003.

TABLE 3.1 Characteristics of Selected Therapeutic Agents in Serum

Molecule	Half-Life in Serum (days)	Therapeutic Concentration in Serum (molar)
Monoclonal antibodies	20	7×10^{-8}
Antiviral agents	0.1	4×10^{-6}
Antibiotics	0.1–0.2	$6 \times 10^{-5} – 6 \times 10^{-6}$
Natural steroids	0.1	$10^{-7} – 10^{-9}$
Contraceptive progestins (synthetic steroids)	0.3–0.6	10^{-9}

SOURCE: Kevin Whaley, director of Antibody Discovery at Epicyte, in a presentation at the International Symposium on New Frontiers in Contraceptive Research, Washington, DC, July 15-16, 2003; Fotherby and Caldwell, 1994; Zeitlin et al., 2000.

Contraceptive antibodies and antibodies directed against pathogens that cause STIs could both be delivered in a number of alternative formulations. For example, gels may be effective, since the antibodies diffuse freely out of gels and into the cervical mucus. Another mode of delivery is antibody-containing tablets, which could be administered vaginally 12 to 24 hours before intercourse. Controlled-release polymers offer another opportunity for long-term protection. Animal experiments with herpes virus antibodies in an ethylene–vinyl acetate copolymer demonstrated that the antibodies offered the animals 100 percent protection against infection with the virus 3 to 7 days after insertion of the polymer (Zeitlin et al., 1998).

Mass Production

However, more effective and more efficient ways of mass-producing antibodies and other therapeutic proteins are necessary to optimize the development of proteins as cost-effective approaches to contraceptive therapy. Current production methods generally entail large-scale culture of cells, followed by purification of the desired protein, which is expensive and technically challenging (Alper, 2003; reviewed by Fitzgerald, 2003). Despite these challenges, scientists are devoting significant efforts to develop new ways of producing pharmaceutical proteins, such as the use of transgenic plants and animals, to reduce costs and to help meet the rising demand.

For example, several companies are working with a number of plant species to develop transgenic plants that produce proteins of interest in large quantities. Plant-based production could potentially decrease manufacturing costs four- to fivefold over the costs of traditional cell culture-based methods (Fitzgerald, 2003). Other potential advantages of this approach over traditional methods include higher product yields and the ease with which production can be increased. Plant-based production would also reduce the risk of contamination with the mammalian pathogens or bacterial endotoxins that may be present in cultured cells.

Nonetheless, plant-based production has a unique set of challenges as well. Potential contamination with residual pesticides, herbicides, or toxic plant metabolites must be eliminated. Plants may also produce proteins with abnormal patterns of glycosylation (addition of sugar chains), which could be problematic for proteins whose structural integrity, activity, and efficacy depend on the human version of glycosylation. In addition, plant glycoproteins contain some sugars that are not found in humans, so there may be some potential for allergic reactions. Moreover, some sectors of society are strongly opposed to the cultivation of genetically modified field crops. For instance, some are concerned that the transgenes could spread in the environment. However, scientists are pursuing a variety of methods that should prevent this from happening, and FDA and the U.S. Department of Agriculture are both establishing a growing body of safety guidelines.

In the near future, transgenic animals might also serve as bioreactors for the manufacture of pharmaceutical proteins. A variety of transgenic animal production systems are under development (Houdebine, 2000), with some products already in clinical trials.[3] The production of proteins in transgenic animals could offer several advantages over mammalian cell culture and other more traditional methods of pharmaceutical protein production, including a competitive cost of goods with respect to the price per gram of material and a favorable capital expense structure with respect to both the absolute amount of investment required and the flexibility of the timing of investment. Transgenic animals may also offer the ability to produce biotherapeutics that would not be commercially feasible if they were made in any other system. For example, as noted above, proteins that display the human glycosylation pattern are more biologically active, and animals are better than other production systems at adding the normal human pattern of sugars to finished proteins. Although scientists are working to develop yeast strains that are genetically engineered to produce proteins with glycosylation patterns that are more similar to those of human proteins, to date the efforts have been only partially successful (Hamilton et al., 2003; Service, 2003).

---

[3]See http://www.transgenics.com/products.html (accessed September 2003).

Recently, there has been renewed interest in the potential of using transgenic chickens to produce therapeutic proteins. For more than 20 years, scientists and companies have struggled to develop an effective method for establishing transgenic lines of chickens, but several recently reported successes have rejuvenated optimism in the field (reviewed by Alper, 2003; Mozdziak et al., 2003). At least three research teams using different methods have now demonstrated that they can make transgenic chickens in proof-of-principle experiments. Although none is yet ready to produce an actual pharmaceutical, experts in the field are highly optimistic that it will happen in the very near future. Several small companies are also attempting to produce transgenic chickens that can serve as pharmaceutical bioreactors by producing human proteins of interest.

The production of transgenic proteins in chicken eggs could be very efficient and economical because each hen can lay 250 or more eggs per year at a cost of 5 cents per egg. Each egg contains almost 4 grams of egg white, which comprises only eight different proteins, greatly simplifying the purification process. The final cost of the purified protein is estimated to be about $10 per gram, or two orders of magnitude lower than the cost by traditional production methods, if it is assumed that 100 milligrams of the transgenic protein will be produced in each egg. In addition, commercial chicken flocks are fast and easy to establish compared with either cell culture bioreactors or other transgenic animals, such as goats and cows. Moreover, chickens are already in use as bioreactors for vaccine production, so the process is familiar to FDA and already has precedence for FDA approval.

Approval of Therapeutic Proteins

These potential advances that use recombinant technologies to generate therapeutic proteins need to be viewed in the context of the recent history of approval of this genre of agents. Some 80 recombinant proteins, including many endogenous proteins, have been approved for clinical use worldwide. A recent survey conducted by the Tufts Center for the Study of Drug Development found that approval success rates for recombinant proteins ranged from 23 to 63 percent globally and from 17 to 58 percent in the United States, depending on the class of agent. Importantly, recombinant proteins in the endocrine class (which would include fertility-related products) fared the best (Reichert and Paquette, 2003). Thus, these approval success rates coupled with current research efforts to overcome some of the cost obstacles suggest that recombinant technology will be a significant source of new medicines.

Advances in Drug Delivery

Over the past two decades, many alternative drug delivery systems have been developed; and sales of drugs administered by patch, implant, long-acting injection, topical gel, controlled-release pill, or nasal or lung spray now exceed $20 billion a year in the United States alone (reviewed by Langer, 2003). More recently, scientists have capitalized on advances in nanotechnology, microfabrication, and other technologies to create novel methods for delivering complex molecules in noninvasive ways, such as implantable microchips that can deliver drugs precisely and on schedule and ultrasound or electrical pulses to force drugs through the skin painlessly (Langer, 2003; Perkel, 2003). Today, 350 companies are devoted to drug delivery,[4] and university laboratories as well as traditional pharmaceutical firms are also conducting research.

In the case of contraceptive development, researchers have thus far focused primarily on controlled-release forms of drug delivery.[5] A major goal of controlled-release drug delivery is to overcome two main challenges: user compliance and side effects. That is, people forget to take pills, and drug levels oscillate with each dose even if they do remember. Controlled-release approaches aim to maintain a steady concentration of the drug in blood, that is, within a "therapeutic window," below which the particular medication is ineffective but above which it could potentially be toxic, while avoiding the need for frequent administration.

Controlled release often entails the release of drug from a polymer, which may be either nondegradable or degradable. The device design can be a reservoir system, in which the drug is encased in a polymer membrane and released by diffusion, or a matrix system, in which the drug and polymer together form a matrix. The rate of release is essentially a function of four variables: surface area, concentration difference, diffusion coefficient, and device thickness. These can be adjusted to control the diffusion of the drug. The challenge is to design an appropriate polymer system that will retain a given drug but still allow it to diffuse slowly, which is a delicate balancing act. An ideal controlled-release system achieves a constant release of drug at the appropriate dose over an extended period of time (days, weeks, months, or even years).

Current controlled-release methods for contraception include implants, long-acting injectables, patches, and devices such as vaginal rings and the Mirena intrauterine device (IUD), all of which deliver steroid hormones.

---

[4]Thomas R. Tice, Ph.D., Southern Research Institute, in a presentation at the International Symposium on New Frontiers in Contraceptive Research, Washington, DC, July 15-16, 2003.

[5]Camilla Santos, Ph.D., Spherics, Inc., in a presentation at the International Symposium on New Frontiers in Contraceptive Research, Washington, DC, July 15-16, 2003.

Controlled-release strategies are increasingly used, however, for a wide variety of drugs, ranging in form from traditional small-molecule drugs to macromolecules, such as proteins.[6] Many delivery routes are being pursued, including oral, intravenous, intramuscular, subcutaneous, transdermal, pulmonary, nasal, buccal (via the tissues of the mouth), ocular, and vaginal. Novel approaches for administering drugs via these routes include:

- Mechanical devices, such as pumps
- Chemical pumps
- Biosensors
- Needle-less devices
- Gels
- Polymer systems, such as microparticles, fibers, films, and coatings
- Nanoparticles to enhance solubility or specificity
- Low-molecular-weight excipients (drug vehicles), such as lipids
- Drug solutions and drug suspensions
- Chemical reactions

In the future, responsive or "smart" materials may also prove useful for drug delivery or as barrier methods (e.g., tubal or vas occlusion). For example, environmentally sensitive materials that respond to the temperature or pH of their environment could be triggered by exposure to semen or other environmental factors (Jeonga and Gutowska, 2002; Qiu and Park, 2001; Rossoa et al., 2003). Temperature-sensitive systems are based on either polymer–water interactions alone or polymer–polymer interactions coupled with polymer–water interactions. Polymers that exhibit a lower critical solution temperature (LCST), such as N-alkyl acrylamide homopolymers and copolymers, shrink as the temperature is increased past the LCST. This LCST is often quite close to body temperature so small physiological changes in temperature may be used to initiate drug release. Bioactive agents may be immobilized or incorporated on or within these systems to allow selective activity of drugs, enzymes, or antibodies. Some progress in the application of polymers to mechanical/chemical contraception has been made in recent years by using styrene maleic anhydride for occlusion of the vas deferens, but the clinical efficacy and lack of toxicity of this polymer have yet to be confirmed (Gupta, 2003; Mishra et al., 2003).

---

[6]Mark A. Tracey, Ph.D., Alkermes, Inc., in a presentation at the International Symposium on New Frontiers in Contraceptive Research, Washington, DC, July 15-16, 2003.

Polymers that can change their structure on the basis of the pH of their environment contain weakly acidic or basic groups in the polymeric backbone, which causes the polymer to swell or shrink with changes in pH. Polyacidic polymers collapse at low pH but swell with increasing pH though the polymer's pK_a.[7] Polybasic polymers exhibit the opposite behavior. Polymers that usually show this sort of behavior are polyacrylic and polymethacrylic systems.

No single drug delivery technology will work for all applications. The chemical and physical properties of the drugs as well as the desired dose and duration must all be taken into consideration when choosing or designing a drug delivery system. Some of the major challenges to be overcome include formulation stability (during manufacturing, on the shelf, and in vivo), achievement of a desirable pharmacokinetic profile, product scale-up and reproducibility, and regulatory issues (especially when new materials are used).

Advances in Biomedical Imaging and Their Application to Contraception

Just as image-guided therapies are gaining favor in reproductive medicine (e.g., in the treatment of fibroids), advances in medical imaging could facilitate contraceptive research and development. Powerful imaging technologies such as magnetic resonance imaging (MRI) have been used to assess the functions of contraceptives in the development process. For instance, the location, migration, and duration of a contraceptive gel or barrier device before and after intercourse can be examined by MRI (Barnhart et al., 2001; Pretorius et al., 2002a, b). In the future, other materials delivered with the assistance of imaging may also play a role in contraception. For example, magnetic substances could be designed as less invasive means of blocking the fallopian tube or vas deferens.

STRATEGIES TO FACILITATE CONTRACEPTIVE PRODUCT DEVELOPMENT

Discovery of Compounds That Modulate Contraceptive Targets

Bridging the juncture between fundamental screens and the initial steps in contraceptive drug development requires special insight and significant risk taking to select the targets for the next and most costly evalu-

---

[7]pKa is the negative logarithm of Ka, the acid ionization constant, which measures the ability of a compound to donate a proton (H+) in aqueous media.

ations. Drug discovery in the field of contraceptive development has several rate-limiting aspects. The identification of specific novel and validated mechanisms to be targeted for drug discovery has been aided by revolutions in molecular genetics, genomics, and proteomics, but the establishment and pursuit of priorities among these many possible targets remain challenges. In addition, the development of lead molecules, once such molecules have been identified, is as important as target identification in the drug discovery process. The unique aspects of the development of protein therapeutics were discussed above. Research in contraception also involves (1) the identification of promising low-molecular-weight lead molecules, which involves high-throughput screening of useful, available chemical libraries; (2) the ability to turn a lead compound into an approvable drug, which demands the use of integrative whole-animal biological expertise to evaluate the efficacy, bioavailability, pharmacokinetics, and toxicities of lead compounds; and (3) the availability of a coordinated and integrated scientific effort focused on contraceptive research. The safety of any new contraceptive agent is of paramount importance, since these agents are used by otherwise healthy individuals. The potential for birth defects if the contraceptive drug fails to prevent pregnancy is also a concern. Thus, contraceptive research faces special and numerous challenges.

To develop new generations of contraceptives, it is important not only to accelerate target identification but also to improve the means of identification of lead compounds that modulate these targets. This might be accomplished first by developing and supporting an infrastructure for high-throughput screening (HTS) facilities and international chemical libraries. Although the pharmaceutical industry has the experience and resources required to accomplish this task, many interested scientists in the public sector lack such experience and resources. In addition, no centralized infrastructure exists to support these activities in the public sector, making it difficult to put into clinical use compounds that modulate validated contraceptive targets. The committee therefore recommends the creation and support of an infrastructure for HTS facilities and the development of international chemical libraries.

These recommendations could be accomplished in a variety of ways. For example, HTS facilities for public use could be developed by a small number of public-sector organizations (e.g., academic institutions) focusing on contraceptive research and drug discovery. The establishment and maintenance of two to four publicly accessible chemical libraries that are useful for contraceptive drug discovery (i.e., by elimination of potentially toxic molecules or metabolically active molecules, identification of potential compounds with noncontraceptive health benefits, etc.) could also expedite contraceptive drug development. One possible concern in setting up multiple facilities is the potential for redundancy. Nonetheless, the establishment of multiple libraries could have many positive implications. For example, maintaining one large library can present a major challenge with respect to sample registration, distribution, and protection, which may be obviated with the use of multiple smaller libraries. Second, scientists could access the library most rapidly able to respond to their request at that moment in time since one location may be too busy to handle all requests expeditiously. Third, through subset searches, chemicals could be eliminated or selected for a second search to minimize redundant evaluation of the same compounds if a second library is used for the second search. Fourth, individual libraries could be tailored to the interest of the institution housing the library so that one library may be more likely to have compounds that are more likely to hit a certain target than another. Fifth, redundancy can be useful in the event that supplies of some compounds are depleted from some libraries. Sixth, competition in library access can help ensure compound quality, which is a major issue with chemical libraries. Thus the availability of multiple libraries should help to foster healthy competition, increased access, reduced bureaucracy, and thereby promote important innovation. All of this should favor a speedier development of new concepts in the field of contraceptive research. The recent experience with the Human Genome Project serves as a prime example of such an interpretation.

The approach taken by the Chemical Genetics Group at Harvard University (Box 3.2) could provide an instructive model for these endeavors. The National Cancer Institute's (NCI's) Rapid Access to NCI Discovery Resources (R·A·N·D) program[8] could also prove instructive for this undertaking. The R·A·N·D program assists academic investigators and investigators at not-for-profit research organizations in the discovery stage of anticancer drug research. The R·A·N·D program can assist in the discovery of small molecules, biologics, or natural products through such mechanisms as the development of high-throughput screening assays, computer modeling, recombinant target protein production and characterization, and chemical library generation. Interestingly, the establishment of a "bioactive small-molecule library" is one of many goals outlined in the National Institutes of Health (NIH) Roadmap,[9] recently put forth by NIH Director Elias Zerhouni as a way to accelerate biomedical research (Zerhouni, 2003). The aim of this program is to involve NIH in drug discovery by developing a library with at least 500,000 synthetic small molecules that could be used to screen potential drug targets. Depending

---

[8]See http://dtp.nci.nih.gov/docs/rand/rand_index.html (accessed October 2003).
[9]See http://www.nihroadmap.nih.gov (accessed October 2003).

BOX 3.2
Chemical Genetics at Harvard University's
Institute of Chemistry and Cell Biology

Chemical genetics involves the systematic use of small molecules to study basic biological mechanisms. In classical genetics, biological pathways are perturbed by mutations in genes. In chemical genetics, in contrast, biological pathways are perturbed by the addition of small, drug-like molecules that affect the function of individual components directly. For example, the enzyme function of a specific protein in a pathway might be inhibited when a small molecule binds to the enzyme active site.

A key technology for chemical genetics is high-throughput screening, in which tens of thousands of molecules are screened in a single day by using laboratory automation. Harvard's Institute of Chemistry and Cell Biology (ICCB), which established one of the first high-throughput screening facilities in an academic setting, provides access at no charge for research groups nationwide (Figure 3.2); these collaborators use a wide variety of assay methods and explore diverse biological pathways from many different organisms (e.g., viruses, bacteria, yeast, fruit flies, fish, and mammals). The ICCB compound collection currently includes more than 250,000 small molecules from a variety of sources, as follows:

- Commercial
  —ChemBridge (66,000)
  —ChemDiv (29,000)
  —Peakdale, CEREP, Bionet, and Maybridge (22,000)
- NCI
  —Structural and mechanistic diversity sets (2,800)
  —Open Collection (110,000)
- Known Bioactives
  —ICCB known bioactives (500)
  —NINDS and Spec+ MicroSource collections (2,000)
- Discrete compounds collected from Boston-area chemists (~1,300)
- ICCB/ICG DOS libraries (>70,000 wells)
- Natural product extracts (marine, plant, fungal; >4,000)

All investigators who deposit data and screening protocols have access to the ICCB results database. The database has safeguards, however, so that the deposit of data into the database does not constitute public disclosure for the purposes of publication or potential patents. Sharing of data and protocols in this way allows comparison of results between screens and has proved valuable for understanding the small-molecule "hits" that are identified as active in each assay. Researchers at ICCB are also developing the ChemBank database to promote sharing of published screening results in the scientific community. Although it is still at an early stage, the ChemBank project will be a freely available collection of data about small molecules as well as resources, including computational tools that can be used to study their properties.

No high-throughput screening projects at ICCB currently target regulators of fertility, but theoretically, the application of chemical genetics to biological pathways important for reproduction could lead to the discovery of basic fertility mechanisms and, ultimately, to the identification of compounds that have potential for development into new contraceptives.

SOURCE: Caroline Shamu, head of screening, Institute of Chemistry and Cell Biology, Harvard University Medical School, in a presentation at the International Symposium on New Frontiers in Contraceptive Research, Washington, DC, July 15-16, 2003. See also http://chembank.med.harvard.edu/ and http://iccb.med.harvard.edu/biology/ (accessed August 2003).

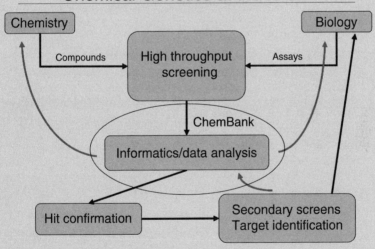

FIGURE 3.2 Overview of the Chemical Genetics program at the Harvard Institute of Chemistry and Cell Biology.
SOURCE: Caroline Shamu, head of screening, Institute of Chemistry and Cell Biology, Harvard University Medical School, in a presentation at the International Symposium on New Frontiers in Contraceptive Research, Washington, DC, July 15-16, 2003.

on how this program is structured, it could potentially serve to meet the needs outlined in the recommendation presented above.

Equally important will be the development of international technological capabilities to facilitate the sharing of data from the high-throughput screens and the chemical compound libraries. Issues related to patenting and legal ownership of ideas, inventions, and compounds will require resolution. Innovative means of partnering that protect intellectual property must be designed with help from the legal community if such a sharing approach is to succeed. Such a shared arrangement of screening and chemical libraries will require the establishment of conventions and standards for intellectual property assignment.

In addition to chemical libraries, consideration should be given to compound discovery through bioprospecting and ethnopharmacologic studies of natural products in developing areas of the world. This approach has yielded a number of valuable drugs and has frequently been used in countries such as India and China, but generally, this approach has been neglected in the United States. This opportunity for international collaboration should be explored.

The next aspect of the drug discovery process requires activities related to optimizing the lead molecule and learning about its effects in animals as well as its bioavailability, biochemical properties, and toxicology. Once investigators in a not-for-profit organization have identified a lead molecule, the drug development process will be accelerated by the sharing of multidisciplinary national and international resources. Historically, this area of drug development has not been well funded or supported.

The committee recommends an increase in the availability of grants specifically focused on activities required to develop novel contraceptive compounds into drugs. For example, NIH could establish a special projects program to fund the development of new contraceptive compounds that offer large potential returns in terms of providing the global community with new contraceptive agents. A recent report on the organization of NIH recommended funding special projects of high risk (National Research Council, 2003), and the development of new contraceptives would fall into that category. An NIH-selected board of reviewers comprising scientists, clinicians, and marketing and business representatives from both the public and the private sectors could serve in an advisory capacity for such a program.

Acceleration of contraceptive drug discovery would also depend on increased participation by the pharmaceutical industry or an increased ability to fund contract laboratories that partner with not-for-profit organizations to make materials and supplies, conduct analytical testing, and evaluate the pharmacokinetic and toxicological properties of lead molecules. Contract laboratories or university-based consortia with appropriate expertise in regulatory requirements could perhaps also perform pharmacokinetic, analytical, and toxicological studies for the public-sector scientists. Funding for such activities is important, as is a mechanism for patenting inventions and sharing in any potential monetary gain.

Finally, expanded Internet use by scientists engaged in drug discovery and development would facilitate interactions among scientists from multiple disciplines and locations, with the hope that greater interactions would lead to the greater sharing of resources for the development of contraceptives. One possibility would be to develop a Listserv consisting of academic, medicinal, analytical, and process chemists, molecular biologists, pharmacologists, pharmacokineticists, genetic and systemic toxicologists, and pathologists who each has a laboratory and an interest in studying specific contraceptive compounds in the ongoing assays performed in the laboratory. Data could be shared among the team members with the goal of patenting inventions and ultimately developing candidates for clinical trials. Alternatively, the development of an Internet site where scientists could pose questions or problems requiring generation of laboratory data on compounds would be useful. Scientists from around the world could access the site to solve particular problems. This approach would require the ability to distribute material to other laboratories for study and data generation; thus, a mechanism would be needed to protect inventions and to share in any monetary gain, should that occur. Legal analysis and input will be necessary to protect intellectual property and patent rights as a motivational force for the work, but it should be feasible to design contracts that are acceptable to both the institutions that own the libraries and compounds and the investigators that make use of them. The NIH is grappling with this issue as it undertakes new initiatives with open access libraries and other resources, and those efforts will likely prove instructive for the endeavors described here.

All of these expanded activities will require additional expertise and an increase in the number of scientists focused on contraceptive research and drug discovery, which could be achieved through endowed professorships or chairs in contraceptive research, new multidisciplinary training grants, and courses or workshops. This topic is covered in more detail in Chapter 5.

Moving Lead Compounds into Clinical Trials

Target discovery research can lead to the identification of molecules with the potential to block the production of functional gametes or a specific stage of the fertilization process, hence showing promise as a contraceptive. Such molecules could be hormonal or nonhormonal in nature. Although the screening of molecule libraries can identify compounds suitable for further testing in studies with animals, many steps must be completed before any study with humans can be conducted. Once a series of molecules has been identified and determined to be effective in a screening model in which a mode of action can be confirmed in vitro or in vivo, a small number of lead compounds must be selected to undergo preclinical testing before phase I clinical trials can be undertaken. The steps in preclinical development to be considered are

- Toxicology studies to establish animal safety before testing with humans;
- ADME (drug absorption, distribution, metabolism, and excretion) studies;
- pharmacological studies of the compound to understand its efficacy;
- preparation of a drug formulation for the desired mode of delivery;
- stability testing to establish shelf life; and
- process chemistry studies to optimally prepare material in quantity.

Without these elements, an IND application cannot be filed with FDA and a clinical program cannot commence. In addition, studies to be submitted in an IND file should be conducted according to Good Laboratory Practice (GLP) and Good Manufacturing Practice (GMP) guidelines (Global Microbicide Project, 2000). The establishment and implementation of GLP and GMP procedures involve considerable time, expense, and training. This "applied" or "translational" research has traditionally been conducted by the pharmaceutical industry, but it is not widely practiced in academic research centers, which may have identified a single promising molecule. In an academic setting, applied research for drug development is not considered attractive from a scientific and career development perspective, and only a very few extramural programs might support it. Most extramural funding programs support basic research and innovative target discovery, and they may also support early clinical studies to demonstrate proof of concept in humans. The challenge is to bridge the gap between early discovery and clinical studies to move promising molecules through these important processes required to administer molecules to humans.

Some small and insufficient laboratories exist at the NIH and in research organizations (e.g., the Population Council and CONRAD), where limited compounds can be tested and further developed. There is also precedence for the effective use of contract research organizations by not-for-profit organizations to conduct the translational research necessary to move lead compounds to a final product. However, for the effective execution of a coordinated development plan, the not-for-profit organization must have in-house staff experienced in preclinical biological evaluation, chemical scale-up, and product formulation and development or easy access to support for such tasks. Currently, financial support is lacking for such an operational structure.

The committee recommends the development and support of not-for-profit-based research organizations offering the know-how, expertise, and tools to complete preclinical studies according to GLP and GMP guidelines, as well as to provide regulatory support for the preparation of INDs and to synthesize and formulate the material needed for initial clinical studies. This objective could be achieved by reestablishing the special projects program (Contraceptive Development Branch) of the National Institute of Child Health and Human Development (NICHD) that was devoted to this process or by creating a new, cross-institutional special projects program in NIH, which would report directly to the director of NIH to fund the development of new contraceptive compounds that offer large potential benefits for the global community. The latter approach may be preferable, as it might allow greater flexibility and speed in the decision-making processes needed to provide funding and to select the most meritorious projects, and is compatible with the NIH Roadmap (Zerhouni, 2003). The P20 exploratory grant mechanism, designed to support planning for new programs, expansion or modification of existing resources, and feasibility studies to explore various approaches to the development of interdisciplinary programs that offer potential solutions to problems of special significance to the mission of the NIH, might also be appropriate for such an undertaking. These exploratory studies can lead to specialized or comprehensive centers. The new program would also benefit from an affiliation with the NIH funded Contraceptive Clinical Trials Network, a group of investigators who are already networked to undertake clinical trials in contraceptive development.

Such a program could perhaps be modeled after NCI's Rapid Access to Intervention Development (RAID) program,[10] which was recently established to assist clinical translation of new anticancer therapeutics that have been discovered in the academic community but for which there is limited interest or capacity for further development in the private sector (Box 3.3). Concerted efforts between private- and public-sector agencies to fund platforms devoted to contraceptive development should be initiated and expanded. Participation by for-profit organizations could be encouraged by specific incentives such as patent life extension, favored tax status, and indemnification for companies engaged in the development of new contraceptives (see Chapter 5).

---

[10]See http://dtp.nci.nih.gov/docs/raid/raid_pp.html#i and http://grants2.nih.gov/grants/guide/notice-files/not98-070.html (accessed October 2003).

BOX 3.3
Overview of the National Cancer Institute's Rapid Access to Intervention Development (RAID) Program

RAID is a program designed to enable the clinical development of promising molecular entities discovered in academic or not-for-profit laboratories but for which the private-sector interest and capacity for further development are limited. The program facilitates the clinical translation of novel, scientifically meritorious therapeutic interventions originating in the academic community by making available to the academic research community, on a competitive basis, NCI resources for the preclinical development of drugs and biologics. RAID helps academic institutions bridge the gap between discovery and clinical testing, so that efficient translation of promising discoveries may take place even in the absence of a capacity for drug development or clinical expertise in the institution where the discovery was made. The goal of RAID is clinical proof of principle that a new molecule or approach is a viable candidate for expanded clinical evaluation, but RAID does not sponsor subsequent clinical trials.

RAID is designed to accomplish the tasks that are rate limiting in bringing discoveries from the laboratory to clinical practice. However, RAID is not a grant program to a particular laboratory. Once a project has been approved, NCI staff interact directly with the principal investigator. NCI contractors perform the RAID-approved tasks under the direction of NCI staff. The tasks that need to be accomplished in any particular case vary from project to project. In some cases, RAID supports only one or two key missing steps necessary to bring a compound to clinical practice. In other cases, it may be necessary to supply the entire portfolio of development

---

New Approaches to Measuring Contraceptive Efficacy

New methods of contraception must offer high levels of effectiveness if they are to be approved by the drug regulatory authorities and if they are to meet user needs. However, measuring effectiveness is not easy. For both ethical and practical reasons, phase I and many phase II studies typically do not use pregnancy as the end point but use a surrogate marker of fertility, such as ovulation (Brown et al., 2002; Rice et al., 1999) or sperm count (Brady and Anderson, 2002). Such markers involve the use of expensive tests, which require skilled investigators and which make huge demands on the time and goodwill of the participants (Croxatto et al., 2002). The mechanism(s) of the method dictate which surrogate marker(s) can be used, and the capacity of the marker to reflect sterility accurately

tasks needed to file an IND. Examples of tasks that can be supported by RAID include, but are not limited to,

- Definition or optimization of dose and schedule for in vivo activity
- Development of pharmacology assays
- Performance of pharmacology studies by a predetermined assay
- Acquisition of bulk substance (under Good Manufacturing Practices [GMP] and non-GMP guidelines)
- Scale-up of production from the laboratory scale to the clinical trials scale
- Development of suitable formulations
- Development of analytical methods for bulk substances
- Production of dosage forms
- Assurance of the stability of dosage forms
- Range-finding initial toxicology studies
- IND-directed toxicology studies, with correlative pharmacology and histopathology studies
- Planning of clinical trials
- Performance of regulatory affairs, so that FDA requirements are likely to be satisfied by participating investigators seeking to test new molecular entities in the clinic
- Provision of IND filing advice

SOURCE: Rapid Access to Intervention Development (RAID) Process and Procedures. See http://dtp.nci.nih.gov/docs/raid/raid_pp.html#i (accessed November 2003).

varies. Azoospermia (Brady and Anderson, 2002) or anovulation (Rice et al., 1999) certainly indicate sterility. In contrast, inhibition of implantation may not be accurately reflected by histological changes in the endometrium (Swahn et al., 1996). At present, there is no surrogate marker that can reliably indicate that the inhibition of implantation has occurred (Croxatto et al., 2001).

The choice of surrogate markers for sterility may be even more challenging for some of the future potential methods of contraception. A method, for example, that impairs the ability of the egg to be fertilized in vitro would be extremely difficult to assess in more than just a handful of women since the retrieval of eggs is invasive and expensive and carries significant risks for the woman. New methods that rely on interfering with much more specific reproductive processes such as oocyte or sperm function may need to use pregnancy as the end point of efficacy studies from an early phase of development. Pregnancy is, however, a relatively rare event, and trials of contraceptive efficacy must involve large numbers of couples for many cycles of use. Such studies are demanding of the participants, are expensive, and tend to overestimate efficacy, since cycles without exposure to the intervention are usually included in the denominator (Trussell and Stewart, 1998).

Trials aimed at demonstrating superior efficacy require even larger numbers of participants at even greater cost in terms of both money and time (Collaborative Study Group on the Desogestrel-Containing Progestogen-Only Pill, 1998). Health care providers increasingly demand good-quality evidence for the superiority of new drugs before they are prepared to purchase and use them. The biological plausibility of better efficacy is not sufficient. Failure to demonstrate superior efficacy jeopardizes the sales of new drugs, reducing the enthusiasm of the pharmaceutical industry to develop them. The development of surrogate markers for unprotected sex might shorten the duration of some studies of barrier methods, which currently require documentation of pregnancy as the end point.

Recent attempts to measure true efficacy in a group of women desiring pregnancy but willing to postpone conception by 1 month (Steiner et al., 1998, 2000) demonstrate the feasibility of an alternative study design that should require fewer participants but that will nevertheless still rely on self-reporting of contraceptive use. Thus, there is a need for more appropriate and novel approaches for the development of new surrogate markers that can be used clinically to assess the potential efficacies of new contraceptive agents and a need to develop new clinical designs to optimize the speed of clinical studies of contraceptives.

Delivery Systems for Future Contraceptives

A key component in the development of any therapeutic agent is the mode of delivery that is selected (i.e., oral, transdermal, transmucosal, subcutaneous, intravenous, etc.; see page 87 for more detail). The particular delivery mode that is ultimately selected is dependent on many different factors relating to the properties of the compound to be delivered, the indication for which that compound is intended, and issues related to acceptability to users.

Irrespective of the sophistication of the science used to identify new molecules, the final product must, of necessity, be simple to use and store, acceptable to the consumer, and above all, safe. This means that delivery systems should be simple and preferably not entail frequent visits to local health clinics or other providers. The more complicated the delivery process is, the more likely it is that compliance will be reduced, and even worse, continuation rates may also be reduced. Complicated dosing regimens, such as ones keyed to particular times in the menstrual cycle, may be self-defeating. In cases in which such timing is critical, the therapeutic agent will need to be present at the appropriate time.

For small molecules, oral pills or, in some cultures, vaginal dosage forms may be the most convenient and acceptable for consumers. However, new delivery systems may have to be considered for new targets that are not easily "druggable" by treatment with small molecules (e.g., for the delivery of peptides of various sizes). For example, it is known that many different chemical entities can be transported across the nasal mucosa or vaginal wall, including small peptides. As described earlier in the chapter, many other approaches for drug delivery are in development, including novel methods for transdermal drug delivery via ultrasound or electrical pulses that may be useful for the delivery of larger molecules.

In anticipation of the identification of new targets and approaches to contraception, as well as the need for dual protection methods (e.g., microbicides administered together with new contraceptive agents), consideration must be given to innovative delivery systems. For example, use of medicated tampons or minipumps placed vaginally could be an effective way of delivering new therapeutic entities while providing the required long-term coverage. Conversely, short-acting vaginal delivery systems such as tablets, films, or suppositories could also be effective, depending on the molecule.

The science of drug delivery systems is constantly evolving and is a technically demanding, highly specialized, and costly endeavor. Although most pharmaceutical companies have entire groups with expertise in delivery systems, only a few academic investigators specialize in this particular applied science. Such factors limit the ability of investigators in not-for-profit organizations to use these technologies in the development of their compounds. The challenge is to establish collaborative efforts between scientists with the expertise and investigators in the not-for-profit sector to develop delivery systems for new generations of contraceptives.

One approach that can be used to meet this challenge would be to establish one or two contract research laboratories that could provide consulting and research services to a scientist who has developed a new compound but who has no way of evaluating the mode of delivery. Pricing in such an environment might be better than if scientists had to seek out their own consultant each time, since the contract company would be assured of business for a finite period of time. Another approach would be to recruit a cadre of ex-pharmaceutical researchers as consultants to not-for-profit institutions. Some of these consultants might provide input by working on a volunteer basis over the Internet or perhaps work for only a nominal fee. A third approach for soliciting broad input through the Internet could be modeled after organizations like Innocentive.[11] This is a company that has been successful in seeking information from the broad chemical community for chemical process improvements and now also seeks input for biology research programs. The program posts problems that need to be solved on the Internet, with specific dollar awards listed per problem (up to $100,000). Involvement with Innocentive may be prohibitive for non-profit institutions, but a free Internet site could perhaps be developed for academic scientists to post problems, where the solver would share in credit and perhaps share financially if the solution is responsible for monetary returns.

Utilizing the power of the Internet would again be helpful in providing scientists information on drug delivery efforts in other research areas, analysis of current delivery systems in the contraceptive field, and contact information for contract laboratories. An Internet site could be established by providing funds to a leading drug delivery researcher in academia to collect and post the necessary information. A fee structure for access to such a site could be established to maintain the site. Free access could be granted to investigators at not-for-profit organizations, while corporate access would be subject to an annual fee. A password access system could ensure the necessary limitations on use of the site.

Engagement of the Pharmaceutical Industry

Given the enormous costs of drug development, the development and testing of novel contraceptives are not likely to be accomplished by government or public-sector programs alone and will require significant participation of the pharmaceutical industry. However, the need for low-cost contraceptives for much of the world presents a conundrum for the pharmaceutical industry because profits from the sale of a new drug would likely be insufficient to cover the development costs. Despite the great need and demand for new contraceptives, the financial incentives for the pharmaceutical industry to develop such products are lacking, and that is the primary limitation to generating interest and action by the industry. The research and development required for a new contraceptive, the long lead time, the multidisciplinary nature of the work, regulatory requirements, and uncertain payoff are likely to be prohibitive—and even with a contraceptive champion within the company, this work can be a hard sell. Incentives to overcome these difficulties are considered further in Chapter 5.

---

[11]See http://www.innocentive.com/ (accessed November 2003).

A number of incentives could be provided to the pharmaceutical industry for the development of new contraceptives for use in developing countries. For instance, some of the FDA processes could be fast-tracked to ensure that contraceptive products being developed for use in developing countries are approved in a timely manner. The patent life could be extended and liability relief could be provided for contraceptive products developed by the pharmaceutical industry for use in developing countries. Cost sharing through the codevelopment of contraceptive products by several pharmaceutical companies or through funding of initial research and development in not-for-profit organizations by the pharmaceutical industry, which would then have first right of refusal, would also be beneficial. Finally, private foundations or government agencies could support the development of low-cost contraceptive alternatives by establishing a central fund that would be supported by governments in those countries that would benefit from such contraceptives. Each contributing country would decide individually how to dispense the products developed. However, this would require a stable commitment of funds to the initiative from these countries and would require the countries to have clear knowledge and to accept that product development could take a rather long period of time (7 to 14 years).

RECOMMENDATIONS

Many promising new targets for contraceptive development have already been identified, and many more will undoubtedly be discovered through efforts to implement the recommendations put forth in Chapter 2. However, validated targets are useful only if compounds can be identified and developed to safely and effectively modulate those targets in humans. The effort will require translational research by a variety of experimental approaches, from in vitro studies through whole-animal studies, to evaluate lead molecules for the purpose of subsequent clinical development. At present, university-based researchers have inadequate resources and information to develop compounds for the most promising targets that they have identified.

Alternative drug delivery systems may also be necessary to accommodate new generations of contraceptives in a cost-effective manner. The science of drug delivery systems is constantly evolving and is technically demanding, highly specialized, and costly. Although most pharmaceutical companies have dedicated groups with expertise in delivery systems, only a few investigators outside of the pharmaceutical industry specialize in this particular applied science. This limits the ability of investigators in not-for-profit organizations to use these technologies in the development of their compounds.

Furthermore, once a lead compound reaches the clinical testing phase, measuring the effectiveness of the contraceptive is a major challenge. For both ethical and practical reasons, phase I and many phase II clinical trials use surrogate markers of fertility, which involve the use of expensive tests, require skilled investigators, and make huge demands on the time and goodwill of the participants. The capacity of each marker to reflect sterility accurately varies, and the contraceptive method dictates which markers can be used. The choice of surrogate markers of sterility may be even more challenging for some of the future potential methods of contraception because they will likely target completely new pathways or steps in reproduction.

Recommendation 4: Implement a mechanism and infrastructure for high-throughput screening facilities and the development of international chemical libraries.

The goal of applying high-throughput drug discovery technologies to all promising contraceptive target molecules or processes could be achieved by supporting a small number of not-for-profit institutions to develop high-throughput screening facilities and chemical libraries. To be successful, the resources and information generated would need to be publicly accessible and shared by the broad research community, with safeguards as necessary to protect intellectual property rights. This may require advice from the legal community regarding intellectual property ownership as it pertains to such a shared infrastructure for compound screening and chemical library development, but the approach taken at the Institute of Chemistry and Cell Biology at Harvard University could provide insight on how to deal with this issue. The establishment of a "bioactive small-molecule library," as recently outlined in the NIH Roadmap, could potentially meet the goals of this recommendation, depending on how that program is structured. The NCI R·A·N·D program could serve as a model.

Recommendation 5: Implement mechanisms to accelerate contraceptive product development and clinical testing once a lead molecule or concept prototype has been discovered in an academic laboratory by sharing multidisciplinary national and international resources.

This objective could be achieved by reestablishing the special projects program (Contraceptive Development Branch) of NICHD that was devoted to this process or by creating a cross-institutional special projects program in NIH that reports to the director of NIH, which might allow greater flexibility and speed in the decision-making processes needed to provide funding and to select the most meritorious projects. Such a program would benefit from affiliation with the Contraceptive Clinical Trials network and could perhaps also be modeled after NCI's RAID program. Existing organizations devoted to contraceptive development play an invaluable role in translational research, but the establishment of new consortia and contract laboratories could further facilitate translational research by providing the necessary expertise for the testing and development of lead compounds. The provision of incentives such as patent life extension, favored tax status, and indemnification to the pharmaceutical and biotechnology industries to expand their contraceptive research and development programs and their collaborative interactions with the public sector would also aid in the development of contraceptives to meet the needs of populations in both developed and developing countries.

Recommendation 6: Develop mechanisms to access, apply, and enhance the technology of drug delivery and formulation science to contraceptive development.

Researchers need to select the best formulation and delivery system for each compound at an early stage of development to minimize development costs. One possible approach is to establish consulting programs in drug formulation and delivery systems that would be available to scientists requiring this expertise. There is also a need to develop novel delivery systems for compounds with unique physiochemical properties (e.g., peptides) and to enable the specific and local delivery of existing and new compounds to a target in the reproductive tract.

Recommendation 7: Develop new approaches to measuring contraceptive efficacy that can reduce the time from phase I and II trials to large-scale clinical testing.

New types of contraceptive targets that entail completely new pathways or steps in reproduction will need new surrogate markers that accurately measure sterility. Work on surrogate markers should proceed in parallel with contraceptive development.

In addition, it would be helpful to develop acceptable new study designs for clinical trials of contraceptives. An example is the testing of contraceptives in women who want to become pregnant but are willing to postpone pregnancy for a month.

REFERENCES

Alper J. 2003. Biotechnology. Hatching the golden egg: a new way to make drugs. *Science* 300(5620):729–730.

Barnhart KT, Stolpen A, Pretorius ES, Malamud D. 2001. Distribution of a spermicide containing nonoxynol-9 in the vaginal canal and the upper female reproductive tract. *Hum Reprod* 16(6):1151–1154.

Brady BM, Anderson RA. 2002. Advances in male contraception. *Expert Opin Investig Drugs* 11(3):333–344.

Brown A, Cheng L, Lin S, Baird DT. 2002. Daily low-dose mifepristone has contraceptive potential by suppressing ovulation and menstruation: a double-blind randomized control trial of 2 and 5 mg per day for 120 days. *J Clin Endocrinol Metab* 87(1):63–70.

Castle PE, Whaley KJ, Hoen TE, Moench TR, Cone RA. 1997. Contraceptive effect of sperm-agglutinating monoclonal antibodies in rabbits. *Biol Reprod* 56(1):153–159.

Collaborative Study Group on the Desogestrel-Containing Progestogen-Only Pill. 1998. A double-blind study comparing the contraceptive efficacy, acceptability and safety of two progestogen-only pills containing desogestrel 75 micrograms/day or levonorgestrel 30 micrograms/day. *Eur J Contracept Reprod Health Care* 3(4):169–178.

Croxatto HB, Devoto L, Durand M, Ezcurra E, Larrea F , Nagle C, Ortiz ME, Vantman D, Vega M, von Hertzen H. 2001. Mechanism of action of hormonal preparations used for emergency contraception: a review of the literature. *Contraception* 63(3):111–121.

Croxatto HB, Fuentealba B, Brache V, Salvatierra AM, Alvarez F, Massai R, Cochon L, Faundes A. 2002. Effects of the Yuzpe regimen, given during the follicular phase, on ovarian function. *Contraception* 65(2):121–128.

Dimasi JA. 2001. Risks in new drug development: approval success rates for investigational drugs. *Clin Pharmacol Ther* 69(5):297–307.

Fitzgerald DA. 2003. Revving up the Green Express. *The Scientist* 17(14):45–47.

Food and Drug Administration. 2003. *FDA Issues Guidance on Pharmacogenomics Data: Guidance Intended to Ensure That Evolving Policies Are Based on the Best Science; Provide Public Confidence in this New Field*. FDA News P03-89. [Online]. Available: http://www.fda.gov/bbs/topics/NEWS/2003/NEW00969.html [accessed December 2003].

Fotherby K, Caldwell AD. 1994. New progestogens in oral contraception. *Contraception* 49(1):1–32.

Global Microbicide Project. 2000. *Global Microbicide Project . . . Responding to an Urgent Need*. [Online]. Available: http://www.gmp.org/ [accessed August 2003].

Gupta SK. 2003. Status of immunodiagnosis and immunocontraceptive vaccines in India. *Adv Biochem Eng Biotechnol* 85:181–214.

Hamilton SR, Bobrowicz P, Bobrowicz B, Davidson RC, Li H, Mitchell T, Nett JH, Rausch S, Stadheim TA, Wischnewski H, Wildt S, Gerngross TU. 2003. Production of complex human glycoproteins in yeast. *Science* 301(5637):1244–1246.

Houdebine LM. 2000. Transgenic animal bioreactors. *Transgenic Res* 9(4-5):305–320.

Institute of Medicine. 1996. *Contraceptive Research and Development: Looking to the Future*. Harrison PF, Rosenfield A, eds. Washington, DC: National Academy Press.

Jeonga B, Gutowska A. 2002. Lessons from nature: stimuli-responsive polymers and their biomedical applications. *Trends Biotechnol* 20(7):305–311.

Langer R. 2003. Where a pill won't reach. *Sci Am* 288(4):50–57.

Mishra PK, Manivannan B, Pathak N, Sriram S, Bhande SS, Panneerdoss S, Lohiya NK. 2003. Status of spermatogenesis and sperm parameters in langur monkeys following long-term vas occlusion with styrene maleic anhydride. *J Androl* 24(4):501–509.

Mozdziak PE, Borwornpinyo S, McCoy DW, Petitte JN. 2003. Development of transgenic chickens expressing bacterial beta-galactosidase. *Dev Dyn* 226(3):439–445.

National Research Council. 2003. *Enhancing the Vitality of the National Institutes of Health: Organizational Change to Meet New Challenges*. Washington, DC: National Academy Press.

Perkel JM. 2003. Nanoscience is out of the bottle. *The Scientist* 17(15):20–23.

Pretorius ES, Barnhart K, Timbers K, Mauck C. 2002a. Use of MRI to determine the in vivo position of a silicone vaginal barrier contraceptive device. *Contraception* 65(5):343–346.

Pretorius ES, Timbers K, Malamud D, Barnhart K. 2002b. Magnetic resonance imaging to determine the distribution of a vaginal gel: before, during, and after both simulated and real intercourse. *Contraception* 66(6):443–451.

Qiu Y, Park K. 2001. Environment-sensitive hydrogels for drug delivery. *Adv Drug Deliv Rev* 53(3):321–339.

Reichert JM, Paquette C. 2003. Clinical development of therapeutic recombinant proteins. *Biotechniques* 35(1):176–178, 180, 182–185.

Rice CF, Killick SR, Dieben T, Coelingh Bennink H. 1999. A comparison of the inhibition of ovulation achieved by desogestrel 75 micrograms and levonorgestrel 30 micrograms daily. *Hum Reprod* 14(4):982–985.

Rossoa F, Barbarisia A, Barbarisia M, Petillob O, Margaruccib S, Calarcob A, Pelusob G. 2003. New polyelectrolyte hydrogels for biomedical applications. *Mat Sci Eng C* 23(3):371–376.

Service RF. 2003. Biotechnology: yeast engineered to produce sugared human proteins. *Science* 301(5637):1171.

Steiner MJ, Hertz-Picciotto I, Schulz KF, Sangi-Haghpeykar H, Earle BB, Trussell J. 1998. Measuring true contraceptive efficacy: a randomized approach—condom vs. spermicide vs. no method. *Contraception* 58(6):375–378.

Steiner MJ, Taylor DJ, Feldblum PJ, Wheeless AJ. 2000. How well do male latex condoms work? Pregnancy outcome during one menstrual cycle of use. *Contraception* 62(6):315–319.

Swahn ML, Westlund P, Johannisson E, Bygdeman M. 1996. Effect of post-coital contraceptive methods on the endometrium and the menstrual cycle. *Acta Obstet Gynecol Scand* 75(8):738–744.

Trussell J, Stewart F. 1998. Contraceptive efficacy. In: Hatcher RA, Trussell J, Stewart F, Cates W, Stewart GK, Guest F, Kowal D. *Contraceptive Technology.* 17th rev. ed. New York: Ardent Media. Pp. 779–801.

Veazey RS, Shattock RJ, Pope M, Kirijan JC, Jones J, Hu Q, Ketas T, Marx PA, Klasse PJ, Burton DR, Moore JP. 2003. Prevention of virus transmission to macaque monkeys by a vaginally applied monoclonal antibody to HIV-1 gp120. *Nat Med* 9(3):343–346.

Waites GM. 2003. Development of methods of male contraception: impact of the World Health Organization Task Force. *Fertil Steril* 80(1):1–15.

Zeitlin L, Olmsted SS, Moench TR, Co MS, Martinell BJ, Paradkar VM, Russell DR, Queen C, Cone RA, Whaley KJ. 1998. A humanized monoclonal antibody produced in transgenic plants for immunoprotection of the vagina against genital herpes. *Nat Biotechnol* 16(13):1361–1364.

Zeitlin L, Cone RA, Moench TR, Whaley KJ. 2000. Preventing infectious disease with passive immunization. *Microbes Infect* 2(6):701–708.

Zeitlin L, Palmer C, Whaley KJ. 2002. Preventing sexual transmission of HSV and HIV: the challenge for active and passive immunization of mucosal surfaces. *Biotechnol Genet Eng Rev* 19:121–138.

Zerhouni E. 2003. Medicine: the NIH Roadmap. *Science* 302(5642):63–72.

4

Improving Contraceptive Use and Acceptability

Decisions about the contraceptive leads that should have highest priority and the delivery mechanisms that should be chosen require more than information on technology and biological sciences. Better understanding of various other factors, such as whether, how, under which circumstances, and by whom a method will be used, should influence whether to begin or continue development of a new contraceptive method. Furthermore, predicting whether couples will use a method consistently and correctly, or whether they will use it at all, requires substantive behavioral research that is performed before as well as after a delivery system is selected.

Even though contraceptive use is an integral part of modern life in most developed countries, at any given time a small proportion of women and their partners who are at risk for unintended pregnancy are not using any method. Studies have shown that in the United States, 7 percent of women at risk for unintended pregnancy were using no method of contraception in any given month. Almost half (47 percent) of all unintended pregnancies each year occurred among these women. The remaining 53 percent of all unintended pregnancies occurred among the 93 percent of U.S. couples who do use methods of contraception, largely because of the inconsistent and incorrect use of effective methods (Alan Guttmacher Institute, 2000; Henshaw, 1998). The same trend has been observed in other developed countries (Larsson et al., 2002; Rasch, 2002).

In less developed countries, pregnancies that result from nonuse and the use of ineffective, traditional methods of contraception are more common (Diaz et al., 1997), for a variety of reasons that include women's attitudes (Brophy, 1990), opposition by husbands (Casterline et al., 2001), lack of knowledge about contraception (Xiao et al., 1999), and rural isolation (Saha, 1994). In a study of 43 developing countries, there was a correlation between a lower number of contraceptive methods available and percentage of married women of reproductive age with unmet contraceptive needs (Benagiano et al., 1999). In 2003, an estimated 705 million women (28.5 percent) in developing countries were at high risk for unintended pregnancy because they were using no contraceptive at all (19.5 percent) or were relying on a traditional method (periodic abstinence, withdrawal, or other nonsupply methods) likely to have relatively high failure rates (9.0 percent). These women accounted for an estimated 79 percent of the 76 million unintended pregnancies that occur annually in developing countries (Singh et al., 2003).

In general, the rates of unintended pregnancy associated with typical use of any contraceptive method (typical use failure rates) are higher than the rates of pregnancy that occur under conditions of perfect use of a method (perfect use or method failure rates). This gap reflects the difficulties that many couples have using their methods of choice correctly and consistently. For example, it is estimated that under conditions of perfect use, no more than 0.1 percent of women relying on combination oral contraceptives (the pill) will experience an unintended pregnancy within the first year of use (Trussell and Stewart, 1998). In fact, however, in the United States, an estimated 7.5 percent of women using the pill have an unintended pregnancy (Ranjit et al., 2001). Surveys of women using oral contraceptives in developing countries indicate that the unintended pregnancy rate is at least 7 percent. This rate is probably higher, however, since many of the unintended pregnancies ending in abortion are not reported by survey respondents (Cleland and Ali, forthcoming).

Contraceptive use effectiveness rates vary widely across sociodemographic subgroups of users, indicating that difficulties in using the available methods successfully are affected by personal characteristics. For example, in the United States, the highest use failure rates among women relying on reversible contraceptive methods were found among those who were under age 25, not in a stable union, poor, and African American (Ranjit et al., 2001). Although some of these differences reflect ongoing disadvantage and resource limitations, others, such as age and personal union status, also reflect differences across stages of women's reproductive lives (Forrest, 1993).

Most women and men spend the overwhelming majority of their reproductive years trying to avoid having children. In the United States, women typically become sexually active at age 17.4, marry at 25.1, have their first child at 26.0, and by age 30.9 have had all the children that they want to have; men in the United States usually have first intercourse by age 16.9, marry by age 26.7, become fathers at age 28.5, and by age 33.2 intend to have no more children (Alan Guttmacher Institute, 2002). These key milestones among men occur slightly earlier in Latin America and the Caribbean and somewhat later in sub-Saharan Africa. Additionally, most men in sub-Saharan Africa continue to want more children until they are into their 50s (Alan Guttmacher Institute, 2003).

Patterns of contraceptive method use differ widely across the world, not only by region but also by couples' reproductive life stages and the desire to space or limit future births (Table 4.1). Women and men who are trying to delay the birth of their first child or to space subsequent births are typically in situations different from those of couples who do not want more children and have different patterns of method use. Women and men in the former group are typically younger.

TABLE 4.1 The Most Commonly Used Contraceptive Methods Among All Couples, Those Seeking to Delay and Space Childbearing, and Those Who Want No Further Births, by Region of the Developing World, Late 1990s and Early 2000s

Region	All Couples	Couples Seeking to Delay and Space Childbearing	Couples Who Want No Further Births
Africa			
Eastern Africa	Injectable or implant	Oral contraceptives	Injectable or implant
Middle Africa	Periodic abstinence	Periodic abstinence	Periodic abstinence
Southern Africa	Injectable or implant	Injectable or implant	Injectable or implant
Western Africa	Periodic abstinence	Periodic abstinence	Periodic abstinence
Northern Africa	IUD[a]	IUD	IUD
Asia			
Eastern Asia-China	Female sterilization	IUD	Female sterilization
China	Female sterilization	IUD	Female sterilization
South-central Asia	Female sterilization	Condom	Female sterilization
Southeastern Asia	Injectable or implant	Injectable or implant	IUD
Oceania-Micronesia	Injectable or implant	Injectable or implant	Injectable or implant
Western Asia	Withdrawal	Withdrawal	Withdrawal
Latin America and the Caribbean			
Caribbean	Female sterilization	Oral contraceptives	Female sterilization
Central America	Female sterilization	Oral contraceptives	Female sterilization
South America	Female sterilization	Oral contraceptives	Female sterilization

[a]IUD = intrauterine device.
SOURCE: J.E. Darroch, tabulations for The Alan Guttmacher Institute (Singh et al., 2003).

A recent study found that one-third of all couples in developing countries who were at risk for unintended pregnancy were trying to delay or space births; among these couples, 56 percent used a reversible modern method, 11 percent used traditional methods, and 32 percent used no contraceptive at all. The other two-thirds of couples at risk for unintended pregnancy are much more likely to be using a contraceptive method: half rely on contraceptive sterilization, 29 percent use reversible modern methods, 8 percent use traditional methods, and 13 percent use no contraceptive. Because those trying to delay and space future births were much more likely to be using no method and because the methods that they did use are typically less effective than contraceptive sterilization, they accounted for 51 percent of all unintended pregnancies in developing countries (Singh et al., 2003).

Thus, although the inherent effectiveness of a contraceptive method is important, the effectiveness of a contraceptive method is ultimately determined largely by whether couples use the method consistently and correctly. In addition to method acceptability, other factors affect consistent and correct use, including those related to the partner, the social and cultural context in which contraceptive use occurs, aspects of the contraceptive method itself, and aspects of the health care delivery system. In short, contraceptive methods must be attractive to potential users, conducive to their ongoing consistent and correct use, and feasible for provision by distribution systems.

It is important to conduct research designed to understand and integrate the views of potential users, their partners, and their providers as early as possible in the development process. In this way, the views of users can influence decisions that must be made over the course of method development to ensure that the ultimate method will best meet user and provider needs. Such information will also be helpful in determining country-specific needs and in crafting the best ways to introduce new contraceptive technology. Funding is scarce for such research in the United States because the projects are often targeted toward clinical application and fail to satisfy criteria for traditional R01-type research grants at the National Institutes of Health, as they are too focused on the product introduction stage to fit into method development budgets, which generally focus on earlier stages of product development. Although the primary purpose of phase I and II is to evaluate safety and to begin testing efficacy, undertaking separate behavioral/acceptability studies before the end of phase II trials is prudent from a resource and market perspective. Such data are generally necessary to secure funding for the large, very costly phase III studies, even within big pharmaceutical companies. To wait until late in the development process and then discover that a new product is unacceptable to a large population is not cost efficient. Knowledge about user preferences early on could perhaps lead to modifications during development that would result in a more acceptable product in the end. Thus innovative approaches to research are needed to predict and increase contraceptive use. There are a number of options for integrating behavioral and operations research into or in parallel with early stage clinical studies so that they will be complementary to the efficient measurement of safety and efficacy. Research in several particular groups of individuals is also of a high priority, as discussed below.

RESEARCH PRIORITIES FOR WOMEN AND MEN

Currently available contraceptives have generally been developed to meet broad safety and efficacy standards. Today, however, there is a growing appreciation of the need to consider contraceptives in the context of various physiological issues that affect women and men at different points in their reproductive lives, as well as in the context of the changing demographics of childbearing. Each of these will affect method appropriateness and acceptability. Therefore, the needs of different groups should be considered and are described below.

Men

Despite the paucity of methods currently available for men (condoms, withdrawal, and vasectomy), men account for a large proportion of current contraceptive users: 17 percent of users in the developing world and 32 percent of users in the United States (Piccinino and Mosher, 1998; Singh et al., 2003). However, the services of family planning providers are oriented primarily toward women and such providers have little experience with providing contraceptive services for men (Alan Guttmacher Institute, 2002, 2003). Moreover, specific safety and biological issues must be taken into account when new methods of contraception are developed for men. The newer hormonal methods in development for men need to take into account both short- and long-term biological effects, as is the case for hormonal methods for women. Effects on the libido will affect men across the life cycle, whereas the potential reversibility of effects on spermatogenesis is likely to vary across the life span. Potential adverse effects related to cardiovascular disease, prostate cancer, muscle mass, and bone loss must also be considered and will affect the acceptability of new methods.

Perimenopausal Women

Because most women and men want far fewer children than would be biologically possible during their reproductive lives, they must use contraceptive methods for most of the interval between the time that they become sexually active and the time that they or their partners reach menopause (Alan Guttmacher Institute, 1995). Thus, women need to continue to use contraception while they are experiencing perimenopausal changes (Gebbie et al., 1995). In much of the developed world, it is not uncommon for women to postpone childbearing until their late 30s and 40s. Thus, women increasingly need to have available reversible methods of contraception for longer periods of time. As shown in Table 4.1, in many regions of the developing world, the contraceptive methods most commonly used throughout the life span are reversible.

Contraceptive methods are used against a background of changing biology and, particularly, changing health risks. For women in their 40s, the increasing risk for fibroids, breast cancer, cardiovascular disease, and osteoporosis need to be taken into consideration when hormonal methods of contraception are used (Glasier and Gebbie, 1996; World Health Organization, 2000). For women in developing countries, where routine health care screening for these conditions is rarely available and where the burden of reproductive disease is enormous, these considerations may be even more pertinent (Elias and Sherris, 2003). New technologies that do not contribute to an increased risk for these conditions, or perhaps even decrease the risk, would benefit these women.

Adolescent Women

Adolescence is typically the time when young people across the world begin to have sexual intercourse, but in the developed world and in many countries in the developing world, childbearing is expected to be delayed until after adolescence (Alan Guttmacher Institute, 1998). Increased attention is being paid to the behavioral vulnerability of adolescents; but, like women approaching menopause, adolescents have certain biological vulnerabilities that present some special challenges, and opportunities, in the development of contraceptive methods for this group. For example, because of their age and stage of physical development, there may be concerns about an increased prevalence of cervical ectopy and its possible relationship to HIV infection. Bone development is another important factor. With increasing worldwide concerns about the nutritional practices and the lack of exercise among adolescents, it is essential that methods not compromise peak bone development. Overall, methods that do not exacerbate these conditions that affect adolescents or that have positive impacts on these conditions would be especially useful for this group.

Many sexually active adolescents are unmarried and have multiple, serial relationships, and some adolescents, especially younger girls, have little power in relationships with older males. There is thus a potential benefit both for short-acting methods that can be used episodically and for longer-acting methods that demand little user input. Methods that provide protection against both conception and sexually transmitted infections (see below) would also be useful for adolescents.

Women, HIV Infection, and Contraceptive Methods

Women infected with HIV have particular needs for contraception. Challenges include limiting the risk of transmission to their partners and to their infants during and after pregnancy. Additionally, decision making about the contraceptive to be used must take into account the impact of the contraceptive on the disease itself, along with any interactions of the contraceptive with other therapies such as antiretroviral drugs or local traditional therapies. However, so little is known about the progression of HIV infection and its relationship to contraception that it is difficult to determine how different contraceptive methods could affect HIV-positive women.

Women at risk for HIV infection have contraceptive needs different from those of HIV-infected women: they need to know how their contraceptive choices will affect their chance of infection in terms of both increased protection and increased susceptibility. They may also want to know the safest means of becoming pregnant without becoming infected if their husband or partner is infected. To date, few studies have assessed the contraceptive desires and factors that affect contraceptive use among HIV-infected and uninfected women. In a sample of HIV-infected and uninfected women in four U.S. states (Wilson et al., 2003), inconsistent condom use was associated with alcohol use, the intention to abort if pregnant, and the belief that a pregnancy would not be upsetting.

The scientific evidence on the effects of contraceptive methods on HIV transmission is limited at present: condom use has been shown to be at least 85 percent effective in preventing HIV infection (National Institutes of Health, 2001), but information on the effects of other contraceptive methods on HIV transmission is limited. A forthcoming NICHD prospective observational study entitled Hormonal Contraception and Risk of HIV Transmission is investigating the hypothesis that hormonal contraceptives may increase the risk of HIV transmission during heterosexual sex, but the evidence is not yet conclusive.[1] No systematic information on the impact of intrauterine devices (IUDs) or other barrier methods like

---

[1]Personal communication, Joanne Luoto, medical officer, Contraception and Reproductive Health Branch, Center for Population Research, National Institute of Child Health and Human Development.

diaphragms or cervical caps on the transmission of HIV infection is available. Furthermore, little is known about whether hormonal contraceptives have an impact on the progression of HIV infection (such studies are ongoing). To address the health and contraceptive needs of the increasingly large group of women at risk for or infected with HIV, the interactions between various contraceptive methods and the risk of both the acquisition and the transmission (sexually and perinatally) of HIV infection must be examined in future studies. Finally, to reduce the risk of unplanned and unsafe pregnancies as well as the burden of HIV disease, direct links need to be established between family planning providers and health care providers for those infected with HIV as well as others with expertise with STIs.

METHODOLOGICAL RESEARCH ON CONTRACEPTIVE USE AND ACCEPTABILITY

New methodological research is needed to develop tools that can better predict the characteristics of contraceptive methods that will be attractive to users in different settings and that will accurately predict rates of use and acceptability. Work is needed to understand the limitations of current approaches and, if feasible, to improve them. For example, current studies may not be tapping all relevant domains that influence contraceptive method choice and patterns of use.

It is not easy to measure the acceptability of contraceptive methods to users, both potential and current (Sundari Ravindran et al., 1997). Acceptability is determined by many factors, including inherent (and often unexplained) preferences regarding particular types of methods, the perceived and actual risks and side effects, and the influences of other people and circumstances in a person's life, as well as how the methods are provided.

Hypothetical acceptability has been used as a surrogate to predict the rates of use of new methods before they are marketed, with research done by organizations such as Gallup/Multi-Sponsor Surveys, Inc., which provide insights into women's stated preferences for contraception.[2] There are no definitive data comparing women's stated preferences with their actual choices or behaviors in using particular methods. In turn, uptake and continuation rates have traditionally been used as surrogates for the acceptability of existing methods. This approach is simplistic. Couples

---

[2]Multi-Sponsor Surveys, Inc., which conducts the Gallup syndicated studies under a license agreement with The Gallup Organization.

may use a particular method not because they like it especially but because it may be "the best of a bad lot." For example, a recent study on contraceptive acceptability, choice, and use found that neither hypothetical acceptability nor conventional measures of acceptability predicted use (Minnis et al., 2003).

Acceptability should be measured across different subgroups of potential users because, although some methods may be very attractive to particular subgroups of women and men, they may not become widely used, and research can identify why this is the case. A survey of U.S. women about their potential interest in using a vaginal microbicide found widely varying levels of interest depending on both the characteristics of the women, especially their potential risk for STIs or HIV infection, and the possible characteristics of the microbicide, including its effectiveness in preventing STIs and HIV infection and its cost (Darroch and Frost, 1999). Also in the United States, women using IUDs have typically reported higher levels of satisfaction with the method than women using other contraceptives (Forrest and Fordyce, 1993); but fear of the method, lack of familiarity with it, and provider reluctance to recommend IUDs have resulted in very low levels of IUD use (Hubacher, 2002; Piccinino and Mosher, 1998).

Methodological approaches that assess the importance of various characteristics of contraceptive methods to potential or current users as well as their perceptions of how different methods rank in terms of such characteristics may be useful to determine their value for prediction of future rates of use (Severy, 1999; Severy and McKillop, 1990; Silverman et al., 1987; Tanfer et al., 2000). Methodologies developed in other fields might also be used to improve the predictive value of early research on method use and acceptability. One example is shared decision analysis tools developed to help people understand the risks, benefits, and implications of alternative surgical choices for medical care in the context of their personal situations and preferences (O'Connor et al., 2003). Recent work by Daniel Gilbert and George Loewenstern aims to provide insight into the cognitive mechanisms involved in predicting future satisfaction among various options (Gertner, 2003). They found, for example, that people were better able to predict their future happiness when choosing an option if they were informed about other people's experience with the option.

People's views of the consequences (costs and benefits) of contraceptive method use are affected not only by their goals regarding pregnancy prevention and their perceptions of side effects and other characteristics of a particular method but also by social factors, including attitudes and beliefs tied to a particular social environment, such as religious upbringing and the expectations of partners, peers, or family members (Raine et al., 2003). In some cultures, the characteristics of certain methods, such as amenorrhea, breakthrough bleeding, touching of the genitals, moistness, and lubrication, make particular methods unattractive (Ladipo and Konje, 1999).

How methods are provided can also be important to their acceptability and to the users' comfort and skill in using them. For example, women who have been counseled about the probability of certain side effects associated with particular methods, such as amenorrhea from some progestin-only methods, are more likely to continue use of the method than those who were not prepared for them (Lei et al., 1996) .

In addition, the importance of the male partner's preference with regard to both pregnancy and the method of contraception has been highlighted in many studies (Alan Guttmacher Institute, 2002, 2003; Mbizvo and Adamchak, 1991; Zotti and Siegel, 1995) that have shown the strong effect of male partners' attitudes on women's contraceptive choice and use. Research with couples is another area needing support to improve the methodologies and research techniques for evaluating the acceptabilities of contraceptive methods. One limitation is the greater level of resources required to obtain data from partners, especially unmarried partners. Another is the question of how to measure and determine the consequences of disagreements between partners regarding family planning and contraceptive use. Additionally, research has not fully captured determinants of acceptability that predict or influence the long-term consistent and correct use of any user-controlled contraceptive method.

The preventive and elective nature of contraception—as well as the high costs of contraceptive development (see Chapter 5) relative to the modest monetary return potential of the contraceptive market compared with that of the market for medications used to treat chronic diseases—suggests the need for a paradigm shift to advance the field. That is, another important frontier in contraceptive development should be the determination of more accurate measures of acceptability and potential use. Once developed, these measures would be most valuable when applied early in the research and development process so that a "go" or "no go" decision about continued development is made before the expenditure of resources for a method that lacks consumer and provider appeal. Moreover, if a "go" decision for continued drug or device development ensues on the basis of a predicted level of acceptability, the characteristics of a method can be market tested with diverse populations when phase II and phase III trials are being conducted. The information gained in such a process can then drive faster and more efficient implementation and delivery of the method (see the section on operations research on page 119). Acceptability research, as described above, can serve as a guide for offering a method in such a way as to enhance uptake and rates of use.

RISK BEHAVIORS AND PERCEPTIONS OF RISK

Contraceptive use has some important similarities to other behaviors, such as cigarette smoking and seat belt use, which provide potentially useful research and public health models for successful risk reduction. Research on risk taking and risk reduction has identified the importance of social, economic, and demographic differences in risk behaviors. These include the strong role of social and economic disadvantage in promoting risk taking, not only because of barriers that limit access to care but also because of the lack of assurance that avoiding outcomes such as unintended pregnancy will be effective toward bettering lives (Darroch et al., 2001). Research regarding contraceptive use and risk taking should pay attention not only to personal factors but also to influences within the relationship, family, and community.

Attention should also be given not only to factors that influence risk but also to their wider causes. For example, research in the United States has shown that good education programs on sexuality can be effective in reducing sexual risk taking among young people, primarily by decreasing multiple sexual partners and increasing contraceptive use. In contrast, the few adequate studies of education programs that focus solely on abstinence have shown that such programs have little, if any, effect on postponing sexual involvement (Frost and Forrest, 1995; Kirby, 2001). Nevertheless, substantial funding in the United States has been directed toward educational programs that promote abstinence and that bar the provision of any information about contraception or condom use except to emphasize their failure rates (Dailard, 2002; Landry et al., 2003).

On the other hand, in 1975 Sweden changed its compulsory sex education curriculum so that it no longer explicitly recommends that sexual activity take place only within marriage and no longer solely promotes abstinence. This revision in the curriculum was accompanied by the establishment of special youth clinics, which provide easy access to contraception. In addition, Sweden's abortion law was revised to allow abortion without charge (Santow and Bracher, 1999). Since these changes were adopted, Sweden has experienced an increase in the number of adolescents using highly effective forms of contraception and a decline in the abortion rate that is unparalleled in the United States and most other developed and developing countries (Darroch et al., 2001; Santow and Bracher, 1999).

These examples highlight the need for more effective ways to inform the public and policy makers about research findings in this area of risk behaviors to promote policy that is congruent with effective contraceptive use. In the seat belt and cigarette examples mentioned earlier, broad-based public education backed by supportive public policy enabled massive behavioral changes. Sweden has shown that the same approach is effective in encouraging behavioral shifts toward more effective contraceptive use and less reliance on abortion.

Research on risk-taking behaviors is equally relevant to women beyond adolescence who either deny or fail to recognize the risks of pregnancy associated with inconsistent or ineffective contraceptive use and thus do not act on them (Jones et al., 2002). In addition, research is needed to study women's perceptions of the chance of becoming pregnant and of the consequences of becoming pregnant, which also affect whether and how carefully contraceptives are used. This is particularly salient among adolescents who may perceive themselves as invulnerable to many risks, including pregnancy (Jay et al., 1989; Trad, 1994, 1999). Further confounding contraceptive use behavior is the fact that for many individuals (primarily teenagers), the consequences of a pregnancy may not be understood (Trad, 1994, 1999), and even if pregnancy is unintended, the consequences may not always be considered a negative outcome (Santelli et al., 2003). In fact, pregnancy may be seen as a mechanism to gain acceptance of friends, the partner, or even family members (Jay et al., 1989).

Furthermore, research is also needed regarding what side effects of the available contraceptive methods raise concerns among different groups of users. While "side effects" are commonly cited as reasons for using no method or for not using certain methods, especially hormonal methods and IUDs, little information is available about what specific effects are most salient to users (Forrest and Frost, 1996).

Because of the focus on the prevention of STIs and HIV infection in the last decade, contraceptive decisions involve not only balancing the benefits and risk of pregnancy but also the potential protection from STIs (see the section on the added health benefits of contraceptive methods on page 122) and thus the perception of sexual risk. The real and perceived risks for STIs are influenced by the partner(s) selected, relationship dynamics, and sexual behavior (e.g., use of condoms).

OPERATIONS RESEARCH ON
CONTRACEPTIVE METHOD DELIVERY

Once a new product is available, the manner in which it is integrated into existing service delivery contexts strongly influences its accessibility and use. In a survey conducted among nonusers of contraception in 13 developing countries, poor accessibility of existing methods was the most predominant reason for nonuse, and this was largely because of a lack of knowledge about existing methods (Bongaarts and Bruce, 1995). A new effort in the United States will survey women to map out the problems that they experience when using methods successfully, to compare these with providers' perspectives, and, ultimately, to better align services to address women's problems with contraceptive use

However, much more research is needed to improve service delivery and thereby foster the successful use of contraceptive methods and to prepare for the appropriate provision of new methods. Details of service provision can be crucial to success or failure in moving from contraceptive method development to contraceptive method use (Bradley et al., 1998; Lynam et al., 1994). For example, contraceptive products that are available only by prescription or that must be inserted by a medical provider must become integrated into the existing medical culture and service delivery contexts. Even in countries where a new contraceptive product may not require a prescription, usual distribution channels still involve interaction with the medical establishment, and clinicians are often sources of information and counseling about nonmedical methods as well.

Certain contraceptive methods require more detailed planning and service delivery adjustments than others. New products or services, such as emergency contraception, sterilization techniques, or the contraceptive vaginal ring, require more than just teaching clinicians about the product or teaching clinicians how to perform the procedure. When a new service or product that is different in design or formulation from existing products is introduced, the entire system must be adjusted so that the new method can be offered efficiently. Interactions between those making decisions about the specifics of method development, method formulation, and delivery systems and those experienced in service delivery can inform these decisions and can provide a foundation for beginning the necessary preparations for appropriate service delivery.

The costs of a new method—those of both the method itself and its efficient delivery—need to be taken into account at an early stage of research and development. A method that is very expensive is unlikely to be widely used, particularly in developing countries. This is especially true for long-acting methods that must be fully paid for to initiate their use. Development of tools and technical assistance for identifying the costs of services and the provision of a new method would help providers, whether they are at a ministry of health level or the clinic level, prepare for new methods.

Providers play a vital role in influencing both uptake rates and the rates of continuation of use of contraceptive methods (Alaszewski and Horlick-Jones, 2003; Edwards, 2003; Espey et al., 2003; Sedgwick and Hall, 2003; Severy, 1999; Thornton, 2003). Provider bias during presentation of contraceptive options is one reason that IUDs and female barrier methods are difficult to access in many countries (Espey et al., 2003; Gupta and Miller, 2000; Johnson et al., 2000; Stanback et al., 1995). In the United States, many women and providers have biases against methods requiring the vaginal administration of a product, and these biases influence consumer demand and consumer acquisition of a vaginally administered product. For example, introduction of an intravaginal ring (NuvaRing) into the United States, where the rates of use and acceptability of vaginal methods like the diaphragm and cervical cap have been very low for many years, offered special challenges. To date, sales are reported to be less than projected. Consumer advertising, education of physicians by the product sales force, continuing medical education programs, and user convenience of once-a-month administration have not translated into the demand seen with other methods used monthly or weekly (IMS Health, 2003a, b). While the level of attention paid to consumer and provider education was similar to most new pharmaceutical products, little attention was paid to service delivery behavior and attitudes or to practices that might enhance consumer use of such products. Research that determines which service delivery practices are important in combating consumer and client biases against vaginally administered methods and that determines the optimal way to increase consumer use of a product is especially important since microbicides (e.g., Buffergel, Savvy, and Ushercell) will probably come to market first as a vaginally administered contraceptive method. Given this prospect, it is important to understand the challenges related to products administered vaginally.

In addition, no one contraceptive method will satisfy all potential users, so the concept of method mix (offering a variety of contraceptive methods with different delivery systems, mechanisms of action, timing of use, and side effects) becomes very important at all program levels (national, state, local, agency, health care site) if individuals are to be able to choose a method that optimally fits into their lifestyle and life stages. With a wider choice of contraceptives, the optimal contraceptive for the individual or couple will more likely be available.

From a programmatic standpoint, it is important to determine how a new method(s) fit into a program's existing method mix. Generally, this decision is made after a contraceptive is approved and is available for use. To offer a new option, these programs may need to drop a method or methods that are part of their current formularies. These trade-offs can be anticipated and should be planned for early—before in-country approval of a contraceptive method. This implies that programmatic assessments of the impact of acceptance of a new delivery system on a program's method mix should be performed soon after adoption of the delivery system is decided, possible side effect profiles have been examined, service delivery requirements have been postulated, and parameters for pricing are known.

Sporadic pockets of service delivery innovations that foster easy access, subsequent method adoption, and correct use will not translate effortlessly into the widespread, consistent, and correct use required for meaningful reductions in unintended pregnancies. Specific program and business efforts designed to facilitate scale-up to broadly accessible programs and to tailor the innovation to local resources are necessary. For any such innovation, identification of a specific service delivery innovation(s) must first occur, followed by testing of the value of the innovation against standard care, before widespread dissemination and then widespread adoption can occur.

Systematic investigation into which service delivery characteristics lead to successful integration of a new product into existing service delivery contexts is a relatively new phenomenon. The insights gained should be built upon through operations research specifically designed to explore which service delivery factors contribute to product access and, ultimately, to successful use of the product by program clients. Formative, qualitative, and quantitative research methodologies are all integral to the operations research needed to inform the service delivery changes that enhance product use.

DEVELOPMENT OF CONTRACEPTIVE PRODUCTS
WITH OTHER BENEFITS

For many individuals and couples, the benefits of contraception beyond pregnancy prevention might influence uptake and encourage more consistent and effective use. Current methods have many well-recognized benefits. Existing combined hormonal methods improve menstrual bleeding patterns (Belsey, 1988; Datey et al., 1995) and can alleviate dysmenorrhea (Milsom et al., 1990), acne (Kaunitz, 1999; Koulianos, 2000), and premenstrual syndrome (Jensen and Speroff, 2000). Increasing numbers of women choose the levonorgestrel-releasing intrauterine system (LNG-IUS) because of the amenorrhea that it confers (Baldaszti et al., 2003; Dubuisson and Mugnier, 2002). Amenorrhea is becoming increasingly acceptable even in many developing countries (Glasier et al., 2003). A recent study in the Netherlands (den Tonkelaar and Oddens, 1999) showed that one-third of young women, given the choice, would menstruate only every 3 months, while more than 20 percent would prefer to have amenorrhea. In a similar way, perimenopausal women appreciate the ability to continue using LNG-IUS through menopause, when it can be used to deliver the progestogen component of hormone replacement therapy (Varila et al., 2001). Because of these preferences of women, a combined pill that can be taken continuously for 3 months without a withdrawal bleed was submitted to FDA and was approved for use in the United States in September 2003 as Seasonale.

The protective effect of combined pill contraceptive methods on ovarian cancer (World Health Organization, 1992) and endometrial cancer (Beral et al., 1999) is perceived as an advantage by providers and enhances continuation rates among well-informed women (Rosenberg et al., 1998). A contraceptive method which actually reduced the risk of breast cancer (Pike and Spicer, 2000; Spicer and Pike, 2000; Ursin et al., 1994) would be enormously attractive to large numbers of women. For young people, the attraction of contraception may be increased if contraceptive use became fashionable (through energetic marketing campaigns) or if it conferred cosmetic benefits such as reducing acne or weight gain.

The development of drugs with two mechanisms and optimizing a single compound for both mechanisms is complex and time-consuming, so the task of developing products that have contraceptive and non-contraceptive effects will be challenging, both synthetically and clinically, but it is an achievable and worthy goal. Alternatively, researchers in the field of contraceptives should consider the potential positive impact that side effects can have on usage as they focus on developing new methods of contraception. The research agenda outlined in Chapters 2 and 3 of this report, however, focuses on highly specific targets (with the exception of dual-action microbicides and contraceptives; see below) with the hope of reducing the side effects of contraceptives. This approach will also undoubtedly limit some, if not all, noncontraceptive benefits (positive side effects). Strategies to combine a new contraceptive with some other agent that prevents a disease might be another more feasible approach to achieve the goal of dual activities in new contraceptive agents/devices.

Similarly, a contraceptive method that also conferred protection against HIV infection or other STIs would also likely be appealing. In a study conducted among college students in California (Holt Young et al., submitted for publication; Holt Young et al., 2002) women indicated that they would be more likely to use a contraceptive method that was also prophylactic for infectious diseases. The need for woman-controlled contraceptive methods that also protect against bacterial and viral pathogens is widely recognized (Butler, 1993; Cates and Stone, 1992; Elias and Heise, 1993; McCormack et al., 2001; Stein, 1992, 1993). Universally, women constitute the fastest-growing category of individuals with sexually transmitted HIV infection (UNAIDS, 2002). In the absence of an effective vaccine or widely available treatment, contraceptive methods capable of preventing sexual transmission of HIV as well as other STIs are crucial for protecting the health of women.

Although the same sexual behaviors put individuals at risk for both STIs (including HIV infection) and unintended pregnancy, a challenge arises because the most effective methods of pregnancy prevention (Swahn et al., 1996) do not protect against STIs, whereas the most effective means of STI prevention (male condoms) are less effective for pregnancy prevention. The result is a trade-off between methods that provide protection against pregnancy and those that provide protection against STIs (Cates and Steiner, 2002; Cates and Stone, 1992). Although one obvious solution to this dilemma is to recommend the use of two methods—one to prevent pregnancy and another to prevent STIs—such an option may not always be acceptable to users; for example, because of cost or factors associated with the use of multiple methods (Cates and Steiner, 2002). Thus, although the need for new methods to decrease unintended pregnancy is important, research to accomplish this objective should not be done in isolation from research to prevent infectious diseases, including HIV infection and other STIs.

Moreover, the addition of a health benefit such as reduced susceptibility to STIs and HIV infection might actually increase interest in using a pregnancy prevention product. In the most recent Institute of Medicine report on contraceptives (1996), the committee clearly spelled out the obvious: unprotected intercourse can result in both unintended pregnancy and HIV infection and other STIs. At that time, the committee recommended that family planning services be integrated into comprehensive programs for reproductive health. The present committee concurs with that recommendation and reemphasizes the recommendation to give high priority to research on new methods that provide dual protection. Nevertheless, it is not always possible to assess the effects of new methods on infectious disease outcomes at the outset of development. Consequently, examination of the effects of new contraceptive methods on STI and HIV transmission should be undertaken in parallel with work on pregnancy prevention. This integration of outcomes might also result in scientific breakthroughs in which the same methods applied to achieve one outcome might be applied to others. Ultimately, the best outcomes will be reached via an integration of research among scientists who work on the prevention of STIs and HIV infection, pregnancy prevention, and even infertility.

Finally, it must be emphasized that although treatment can substantially reduce mother- to-child HIV transmission (National Research Council, 1999), the most effective strategy to prevent mother-to-child transmission of HIV is pregnancy prevention among HIV-infected women, regardless of the effect of such methods on STIs and HIV infection. Issues related to maternal morbidity and mortality among HIV-infected women must also be taken into account in the development of new contraceptive methods, regardless of their direct effect on HIV infection and other STIs.

IMPROVING EXISTING METHODS

As discussed above, research is simultaneously needed to better understand the reasons behind the choice of a contraceptive method and discontinuation of its use and the reasons for gaps in method use and incorrect and inconsistent use. Such factors are likely to affect the uptake of new methods as well as the use of existing, effective methods. Although a number of reversible methods of contraception are available, modern methods fall into only three categories: barrier methods, hormonal methods, and IUDs. All have their drawbacks. Gaps between use failure and method failure rates and differences across subgroups are widest for methods that require greater user involvement and methods over which users have greater control over use and continuation (Ranjit et al., 2001; Trussell and Stewart, 1998). Currently available barrier methods have relatively high failure rates (Cleland and Ali, forthcoming; Ranjit et al., 2001; Trussell and Stewart, 1998), and effectiveness depends on correct and consistent use. The use of such methods is not easy: women relying on male condoms are overrepresented among women having abortions (Jones et al., 2002). Hormonal methods are available in a number of different delivery systems, some of which (e.g., implants) make no demands on compliance. However, the most popular route of administration, oral contraception, relies heavily on compliance for effectiveness (Emans et al., 1987; Potter et al., 1996; Ranjit et al., 2001; Rosenberg and Waugh, 1999; Trussell and Stewart, 1998).

Combined hormonal methods have been associated with a very small increased risk of cardiovascular disease (Beral et al., 1999; Kemmeren et al., 2001; Tanis et al., 2001; World Health Organization, 1998) and of breast cancer (Collaborative Group on Hormonal Factors in Breast Cancer, 1996) and cervical cancer (Smith et al., 2003). In the case of breast cancer, a slight increase in relative risk for breast cancer among women under age 40 has been observed, but the absolute risk is very low because the risk of breast cancer in this age group is so low. When the overall risk of breast cancer across all age groups is assessed, no increase in risk is seen. However, among the various studies undertaken to examine the risk for disease associated with hormonal methods, no single study adjusted for all known confounding factors simultaneously. Thus, the debate as to whether the reported risks are real continues. In any case, if there is a real increase in disease risk, it is very low. Low-dose progestin-only methods are associated with a high incidence of irregular bleeding (D'Arcangues et al., 1992), and IUDs have historically been relatively unpopular in most developed countries (Hubacher, 2002; Oddens et al., 1994).

Continuation rates are not a surrogate for acceptability (Severy, 1999; Severy and Thapa, 1994), and acceptability does not guarantee use (Minnis et al., 2003). Fear of serious health risks and fear of side effects often lead to discontinuation (Grubb, 1987; Larsson et al., 1997) or deter many women from even starting any existing hormonal methods (Svare et al., 1997). Overall, most currently available methods have discontinuation rates approaching 50 percent after 1 year of use, usually because of side effects (Rosenberg et al., 1995; Trussell and Vaughan, 1999). Women who continue using a method often do so despite the side effects, which they are prepared to tolerate in return for pregnancy prevention. Nevertheless, difficulties with compliance and contraceptive discontinuation account for large numbers of unintended pregnancies (Jones et al., 2002; Rosenberg et al., 1995). Indeed, more than half the women obtaining abortions in the United States in 2000 claimed to have been using a method of contraception during the month that they became pregnant (Jones et al., 2002): 14 percent had been using the contraceptive pill, and 28 percent had been using the male condom.

Improvements in efficacy (Rice et al., 1999; Task Force on Postovulatory Methods of Fertility Regulation, 1998) and reduction of the side effects (Task Force on Postovulatory Methods of Fertility Regulation, 1998; Wildemeersch et al., 1999) resulting from the use of existing methods have been made over the last four decades, and new delivery systems have also been developed over that time. Nevertheless, efforts should continue to increase the range of acceptable methods, their accessibility, and their efficacy and ease of use.

RECOMMENDATIONS

To be successful, contraceptive methods must be attractive to potential users and must be feasible for distribution systems to provide. Understanding and integrating the views of potential users, their partners, and their providers early in the development process can influence the course of development and help ensure that the resultant method will meet user and provider needs. There are a number of options for integrating behavioral and operations research into or in parallel with early stage clinical studies so that they will be complementary to the efficient measurement of safety and efficacy.

In addition, the development of contraceptives that provide additional benefits beyond pregnancy prevention would enhance their attractiveness. Current methods offer a number of added benefits, including alleviation of dysmenorrhea, acne, or premenstrual syndrome; improved endometrial bleeding patterns; or amenorrhea. The protective effect of the combined pill on ovarian and endometrial cancer also enhances continuation rates among well-informed women. Thus, contraceptives that reduced the risk of other diseases such as breast or prostate cancer would likely have wide appeal. A contraceptive method that also conferred protection against HIV infection and other STIs is likely to have widespread benefit as well. Moreover, the development, evaluation, and implementation of innovative models of health care delivery that integrate family planning, STI, and HIV infection services could be very beneficial.

Recommendation 8: Provide incentives and mechanisms for the integration of behavioral and operations research, including the views of providers as well as those of potential users and their partners, early in the contraceptive research and development process.

Acceptability is determined by many factors, including inherent (and often unexplained) preferences; the perceived and actual risks and side effects; life stage and whether more children are desired eventually; social factors, including cultural preferences and the expectations of partners, peers, or family members. More accurate measures of acceptability and potential use would be valuable when applied early in the development process to improve decisions about continued development before the expenditure of resources for a method that lacks consumer and provider appeal. New methodological research is also needed to develop tools that can better predict the characteristics of contraceptive methods that will be attractive to users in different settings and life stages.

Providers play a vital role in influencing both uptake rates and continuation rates of contraceptive method use. Thus, research that determines which service delivery practices are effective for increasing acceptance and use of contraceptives would be useful as well.

Recommendation 9: During the development of drugs and drug delivery systems, efforts should be made to discover, enhance, and promote the noncontraceptive health benefits of existing and new methods of contraception. Intensified efforts to develop new contraceptive methods that are prophylactic for HIV infection and other STIs are especially important.

Clinical evaluation and registration of a single product for two indications is more complex and time-consuming, but it is feasible and has been accomplished for some therapeutic agents. Furthermore, several formulations that exhibit both spermicidal and microbicidal effects are now in clinical trials, lending credence to the potential for success in achieving this goal.

REFERENCES

Alan Guttmacher Institute (AGI). 1995. *Hopes and Realities: Closing the Gap between Women's Aspirations and Their Reproductive Experiences.* New York: AGI.

Alan Guttmacher Institute (AGI). 1998. *Into a New World: Young Women's Sexual and Reproductive Lives.* New York: AGI.

Alan Guttmacher Institute (AGI). 2000. *Fulfilling the Promise: Public Policy and U.S. Family Planning Clinics.* New York: AGI.

Alan Guttmacher Institute (AGI). 2002. *In Their Own Right: Addressing the Sexual and Repro-ductive Health Needs of American Men.* New York: AGI.

Alan Guttmacher Institute (AGI). 2003. *In Their Own Right: Addressing the Sexual and Repro-ductive Health Needs of Men Worldwide.* New York: AGI.

Alaszewski A, Horlick-Jones T. 2003. How can doctors communicate information about risk more effectively? *BMJ* 327(7417):728–731.

Baldaszti E, Wimmer-Puchinger B, Loschke K. 2003. Acceptability of the long-term contra-ceptive levonorgestrel-releasing intrauterine system (Mirena): a 3-year follow-up study. *Contraception* 67(2):87–91.

Belsey EM. 1988. Vaginal bleeding patterns among women using one natural and eight hormonal methods of contraception. *Contraception* 38(2):181–206.

Benagiano G, Franceschinis P, Pera A. 1999. Abortion in adolescence. In: Coutinho EM, Spinola P, eds. *Reproductive Medicine: A Millennium Review, The Proceedings of the 10th World Congress on Human Reproduction.* New York: The Parthenon Publishing Group. Pp. 55–62.

Beral V, Hermon C, Kay C, Hannaford P, Darby S, Reeves G. 1999. Mortality associated with oral contraceptive use: 25-year follow up of cohort of 46,000 women from Royal Col-lege of General Practitioners' oral contraception study. *BMJ* 318(7176):96–100.

Bongaarts J, Bruce J. 1995. The causes of unmet need for contraception and the social content of services. *Stud Fam Plann* 26(2):57–75.

Bradley J, Lynam PF, Dwyer JC, Wambwa GE. 1998. *Whole-Site Training: A New Approach to the Organization of Training.* AVSC Working Paper No. 11. New York: AVSC Interna-tional.

Brophy G. 1990. Unmet need and nonuse of family planning in Botswana. *Popul Today* 18(11):6–7.

Butler D. 1993. WHO widens focus of AIDS research. *Nature* 366(6453):293.

Casterline JB, Sathar ZA, ul Haque M. 2001. Obstacles to contraceptive use in Pakistan: a study in Punjab. *Stud Fam Plann* 32(2):95–110.

Cates W Jr, Steiner MJ. 2002. Dual protection against unintended pregnancy and sexually transmitted infections: what is the best contraceptive approach? *Sex Transm Dis* 29(3):168–174.

Cates W Jr, Stone KM. 1992. Family planning, sexually transmitted diseases and contracep-tive choice: a literature update—Part II. *Fam Plann Perspect* 24(3):122–128.

Cleland J, Ali M. *Dynamics of Contraceptive Use, in Levels and Trends of Contraceptive Use as Addressed in 2002.* New York: United Nations, forthcoming.

Collaborative Group on Hormonal Factors in Breast Cancer. 1996. Breast cancer and hor-monal contraceptives: collaborative reanalysis of individual data on 53,297 women with breast cancer and 100,239 women without breast cancer from 54 epidemiological studies. *Lancet* 347(9017):1713–1727.

Dailard C. 2002. Abstinence promotion and teen family planning: the misguided drive for equal funding. *The Guttmacher Report on Public Policy* 5(1):1–3.

D'Arcangues C, Odlind V, Fraser IS. 1992. Dysfunctional uterine bleeding induced by exogenous hormones. In: D'Arcangues C, Alexander NJ, eds. *Steroid Hormones and Uter-ine Bleeding.* Washington, DC: AAAS Press. Pp. 81–105.

Darroch JE, Frost JJ. 1999. Women's interest in vaginal microbicides. *Fam Plann Perspect* 31(1):16–23.

Darroch JE, Frost JJ, Singh S, The Study Team. 2001. *Can More Progress Be Made? Teenage Sexual Reproductive Behavior in Developed Countries.* Occasional Report, No. 3. New York: The Alan Guttmacher Institute.

Datey S, Gaur LN, Saxena BN. 1995. Vaginal bleeding patterns of women using different contraceptive methods (implants, injectables, IUDs, oral pills): an Indian experience. An ICMR Task Force Study. Indian Council of Medical Research. *Contraception* 51(3):155–165.

den Tonkelaar I, Oddens BJ. 1999. Preferred frequency and characteristics of menstrual bleeding in relation to reproductive status, oral contraceptive use, and hormone replacement therapy use. *Contraception* 59(6):357–362.

Diaz S, Zepeda A, Maturana X, Reyes MV, Miranda P , Casado ME, Peralta O, Croxatto HB. 1997. Fertility regulation in nursing women: contraceptive performance, duration of lactation, infant growth, and bleeding patterns during use of progesterone vaginal rings, progestin-only pills, Norplant implants, and Copper T 380-A intrauterine devices. *Contraception* 56:223–232.

Dubuisson JB, Mugnier E. 2002. Acceptability of the levonorgestrel-releasing intrauterine system after discontinuation of previous contraception: results of a French clinical study in women aged 35 to 45 years. *Contraception* 66(2):121–128.

Edwards A. 2003. Communicating risks. *BMJ* 327(7417):691–692.

Elias C, Sherris J. 2003. Reproductive and sexual health of older women in developing countries. *BMJ* 327(7406):64–65.

Elias CJ, Heise L. 1993. *The Development of Microbicides: A New Method of HIV Prevention for Women.* Working Paper No. 6. New York: The Population Council.

Emans SJ, Grace E, Woods ER, Smith DE, Klein K, Merola J. 1987. Adolescents' compliance with the use of oral contraceptives. *JAMA* 257(24):3377–3381.

Espey E, Ogburn T, Espey D, Etsitty V. 2003. IUD-related knowledge, attitudes and practices among Navajo Area Indian Health Service providers. *Perspect Sex Reprod Health* 35(4):169–173.

Forrest JD. 1993. Timing of reproductive life stages. *Obstet Gynecol* 82(1):105–111.

Forrest JD, Fordyce RR. 1993. Women's contraceptive attitudes and use in 1992. *Fam Plann Perspect* 25(4):175–179.

Forrest JD, Frost JJ. 1996. The family planning attitudes and experiences of low-income women. *Fam Plann Perspect* 28(6):246–255, 277.

Frost JJ, Forrest JD. 1995. Understanding the impact of effective teenage pregnancy prevention programs. *Fam Plann Perspect* 27(5):188–195.

Gebbie AE, Glasier A, Sweeting V. 1995. Incidence of ovulation in perimenopausal women before and during hormone replacement therapy. *Contraception* 52(4):221–222.

Gertner J. 2003, September 7. The futile pursuit of happiness. *The New York Times Magazine,* pp. 44–47, 86, 90–91.

Glasier A, Gebbie A. 1996. Contraception for the older woman. *Baillieres Clin Obstet Gynaecol* 10(1):121–138.

Glasier AF, Smith KB, van der Spuy ZM, Ho PC, Cheng L, Dada K, Wellings K, Baird DT. 2003. Amenorrhea associated with contraception: an international study on acceptability. *Contraception* 67(1):1–8.

Grubb GS. 1987. Women's perceptions of the safety of the pill: a survey in eight developing countries. Report of the perceptions of the pill survey group. *J Biosoc Sci* 19(3):313–321.

Gupta S, Miller JE. 2000. A survey of GP views in intra-uterine contraception. *Br J Fam Plann* 26(2):81–84.

Henshaw SK. 1998. Unintended pregnancy in the United States. *Fam Plann Perspect* 30(1):24–29, 46.

Holt Young B, Ngo L, Morwitz V, Harrison P, Whaley K, Nguyen A, Pettifore A, Russel-Fisk E. 2002. *The Market Potential for Microbicides among Young Women.* Microbicide 2002 Conference, Antwerp, Belgium. May 12–15, 2002.

Holt Young B, Ngo L, Morwitz V, Harrison P, Whaley K, Nguyen A. Submitted for publication. *Microbicide Preferences Among College Women in California.*

Hubacher D. 2002. The checkered history and bright future of intrauterine contraception in the United States. *Perspect Sex Reprod Health* 34(2):98–103.

IMS Health, 2003a. *National Prescription Audit Plus, MIDAS for Manufacturer Years 2001 and 2002.* Fairfield, CT: IMS.

IMS Health, 2003b. *Dispensed New Prescriptions (NRX) and Total Prescriptions (TRX), October to December 2002.* Fairfield, CT: IMS.

Institute of Medicine. 1996. *Contraceptive Research and Development: Looking to the Future.* Harrison PF, Rosenfield A, eds. Washington, DC: National Academy Press.

Jay MS, DuRant RH, Litt IF. 1989. Female adolescents' compliance with contraceptive regimes. *Pediatr Clin North Am* 36(3):731–746.

Jensen JT, Speroff L. 2000. Health benefits of oral contraceptives. *Obstet Gynecol Clin N Am* 27(4):705–721.

Johnson L, Katz K, Janowitz B. 2000. *Determining Reasons for Low IUD Use in El Salvador.* Research Triangle Park, NC: Family Health International.

Jones RK, Darroch JE, Henshaw SK. 2002. Contraceptive use among U.S. women having abortions in 2000–2001. *Perspect Sex Reprod Health* 34(6):294–303.

Kaunitz AM. 1999. Oral contraceptive health benefits: perception versus reality. *Contraception* 59(1 suppl):29S–33S.

Kemmeren JM, Algra A, Grobbee DE. 2001. Third generation oral contraceptives and risk of venous thrombosis: meta-analysis. *BMJ* 323(7305):131–134.

Kirby D. 2001. *Emerging Answers: Research Findings on Programs to Reduce Teen Pregnancy.* Washington, DC: National Campaign to Prevent Teen Pregnancy.

Koulianos GT. 2000. Treatment of acne with oral contraceptives: criteria for pill selection. *Cutis* 66(4):281–286.

Ladipo OA, Konje JC. 1999. Barriers to contraceptive use in developing countries. In: Coutinho EM, Spinola P, eds. *Reproductive Medicine: A Millennium Review, The Proceedings of the 10th World Congress on Human Reproduction.* New York: The Parthenon Publishing Group. Pp. 66–79.

Landry D, Darroch JE, Singh S, Higgins J. 2003. Factors associated with the content of sex education in U.S. public secondary schools. *Perspectives on Sexual and Reproductive Health* 35(6):261–269.

Larsson G, Blohm F, Sundell G, Andersch B, Milsom I. 1997. A longitudinal study of birth control and pregnancy outcome among women in a Swedish population. *Contraception* 56(1):9–16.

Larsson M, Aneblom G, Odlind V, Tyden T. 2002. Reasons for pregnancy termination, contraceptive habits and contraceptive failure among Swedish women requesting an early pregnancy termination. *Acta Obstet Gynecol Scand* 81(1):64–71.

Lei ZW, Wu SC, Garceau RJ, Jiang S, Yang QZ, Wang WL, Vander Meulen TC. 1996. Effect of pretreatment counseling on discontinuation rates in Chinese women given depomedroxyprogesterone acetate for contraception. *Contraception* 53(6):357–361.

Lynam PF, Dwyer JC, Bradley J. 1994. *Inreach: Reaching Potential Family Planning Clients within Health Institutions.* AVSC Working Paper No. 5. New York: AVSC International.

Mbizvo MT, Adamchak DJ. 1991. Family planning knowledge, attitudes, and practices of men in Zimbabwe. *Stud Fam Plann* 22(1):31–38.

McCormack S, Hayes R, Lacey CJ, Johnson AM. 2001. Microbicides in HIV prevention. *BMJ* 322(7283):410–413.

Milsom I, Sundell G, Andersch B. 1990. The influence of different combined oral contraceptives on the prevalence and severity of dysmenorrhea. *Contraception* 42(5):497–506.

Minnis AM, Shiboski SC, Padian NS. 2003. Barrier contraceptive method acceptability and choice are not reliable indicators of use. *Sex Transm Dis* 30(7):556–561.

National Institutes of Health. 2001. *Scientific Evidence on Condom Effectiveness for Sexually Transmitted Disease (STD) Prevention.* [Online]. Available: http://www.niaid.nih.gov/dmid/stds/condomreport.pdf, page 17 [accessed November 2003].

National Research Council. 1999. *Reducing the Odds: Preventing Perinatal Transmission of HIV in the United States.* Stoto MA, Almario DA, McCormick MC, eds. Washington, DC: National Academy Press.

O'Connor AM, Legare F, Stacey D. 2003. Risk communication in practice: the contribution of decision aids. *BMJ* 327(7417):736–740.

Oddens BJ, Visser AP, Vemer HM, Everaerd WT, Lehert P. 1994. Contraceptive use and attitudes in Great Britain. *Contraception* 49(1):73–86.

Piccinino LJ, Mosher WD. 1998. Trends in contraceptive use in the United States: 1982–1995. *Fam Plann Perspect* 30(1):4–10, 46.

Pike MC, Spicer DV. 2000. Hormonal contraception and chemoprevention of female cancers. *Endocr Relat Cancer* 7(2):73–83.

Potter L, Oakley D, de Leon-Wong E, Canamar R. 1996. Measuring compliance among oral contraceptive users. *Fam Plann Perspect* 28(4):154–158.

Raine T, Minnis AM, Padian NS. 2003. Determinants of contraceptive method among young women at risk for unintended pregnancy and sexually transmitted infections. *Contraception* 68(1):19–25.

Ranjit N, Bankole A, Darroch JE, Singh S. 2001. Contraceptive failure in the first two years of use: differences across socioeconomic subgroups. *Fam Plann Perspect* 33(1):19–27.

Rasch V. 2002. Contraceptive failure: results from a study conducted among women with accepted and unaccepted pregnancies in Denmark. *Contraception* 66(2):109–116.

Rice CF, Killick SR, Dieben T, Coelingh Bennink H. 1999. A comparison of the inhibition of ovulation achieved by desogestrel 75 micrograms and levonorgestrel 30 micrograms daily. *Hum Reprod* 14(4):982–985.

Rosenberg M, Waugh MS. 1999. Causes and consequences of oral contraceptive non-compliance. *Am J Obstet Gynecol* 180(2 Pt 2):276–279.

Rosenberg MJ, Waugh MS, Long S. 1995. Unintended pregnancies and use, misuse and discontinuation of oral contraceptives. *J Reprod Med* 40(5):355–360.

Rosenberg MJ, Waugh MS, Burnhill MS. 1998. Compliance, counseling and satisfaction with oral contraceptives: a prospective evaluation. *Fam Plann Perspect* 30(2):89–92, 104.

Saha TD. 1994. Community resources and reproductive behaviour in rural Bangladesh. *Asia Pac Popul J* 9(1):3–18.

Santelli J, Rochat R, Hatfield-Timajchy K, Gilbert BC, Curtis K, Cabral R, Hirsch JS, Schieve L. 2003. The measurement and meaning of unintended pregnancy. *Perspect Sex Reprod Health* 35(2):94–101.

Santow G, Bracher M. 1999. Explaining trends in teenage childbearing in Sweden. *Stud Fam Plann* 30(3):169–182.

Sedgwick P, Hall A. 2003. Teaching medical students and doctors how to communicate risk. *BMJ* 327(7417):694–695.

Severy LJ. 1999. Acceptability as a critical component of clinical trials. *Adv Pop* 3:103–122.

Severy LJ, McKillop K. 1990. Low-income women's perceptions of family planning service alternatives. *Fam Plann Perspect* 22(4):150–157, 168.

Severy LJ, Thapa S. 1994. Preferences and tolerance as determinants of contraceptive acceptability. *Adv Pop* 2:119–139.

Silverman J, Torres A, Forrest JD. 1987. Barriers to contraceptive services. *Fam Plann Perspect* 19(3):94–97, 101–102.

Singh S, Darroch JE, Vlassoff M, Nadeau J. 2003. *Adding It Up: The Benefits of Investing in Sexual and Reproductive Health Care*. New York: The Alan Guttmacher Institute.

Smith JS, Green J, Berrington de Gonzalez A, Appleby P, Peto J, Plummer M, Franceschi S, Beral V. 2003. Cervical cancer and use of hormonal contraceptives: a systematic review. *Lancet* 361(9364):1159–1167.

Spicer DV, Pike MC. 2000. Future possibilities in the prevention of breast cancer: luteinizing hormone-releasing hormone agonists. *Breast Cancer Res* 2(4):264–267.

Stanback J, Omondi-Odhiambo, Omuodo D. 1995. *Why Has IUD Use Slowed in Kenya? Part A: Qualitative Assessment of IUD Service Delivery in Kenya. Final Report*. Research Triangle Park, NC: Family Health International.

Stein Z. 1993. HIV prevention: an update on the status of methods women can use. *Am J Public Health* 83(10):1379–1382.

Stein ZA. 1992. The double bind in science policy and the protection of women from HIV infection. *Am J Public Health* 82(11):1471–1472.

Sundari Ravindran TK, Berer M, Cottingham J, eds. 1997. *Beyond Acceptability: Users' Perspectives on Contraception*. Geneva: World Health Organization.

Svare EI, Kjaer SK, Poll P, Bock JE. 1997. Determinants for contraceptive use in young, single, Danish women from the general population. *Contraception* 55(5):287–294.

Swahn ML, Westlund P, Johannisson E, Bygdeman M. 1996. Effect of post-coital contraceptive methods on the endometrium and the menstrual cycle. *Acta Obstet Gynecol Scand* 75(8):738–744.

Tanfer K, Wierzbicki S, Payn B. 2000. Why are US women not using long-acting contraceptives? *Fam Plann Perspect* 32(4):176–183, 191.

Tanis BC, van den Bosch MA, Kemmeren JM, Cats VM, Helmerhorst FM, Algra A, van der Graaf Y, Rosendaal FR. 2001. Oral contraceptives and the risk of myocardial infarction. *N Engl J Med* 345(25):1787–1793.

Task Force on Postovulatory Methods of Fertility Regulation. 1998. Randomised controlled trial of levonorgestrel versus the Yuzpe regimen of combined oral contraceptives for emergency contraception. *Lancet* 352(9126):428–433.

Thornton H. 2003. Patients' understanding of risk. *BMJ* 327(7417):693–694.

Trad PV. 1994. Developmental previewing: enhancing the adolescent's predictions of behavioral consequences. *J Clin Psychol* 50(6):814–829.

Trad PV. 1999. Assessing the patterns that prevent teenage pregnancy. *Adolscence* 34(133):221–240.

Trussell J, Stewart F. 1998. Contraceptive efficacy. In: Hatcher RA, Trussell J, Stewart F, Cates W, Stewart GK, Guest F, Kowal D, eds. *Contraceptive Technology*. 17th rev. ed. New York: Ardent Media.

Trussell J, Vaughan B. 1999. Contraceptive failure, method-related discontinuation and resumption of use: results from the 1995 National Survey of Family Growth. *Fam Plann Perspect* 31(2):64–72, 93.

UNAIDS (Joint United Nations Program on HIV/AIDS). 2002. *AIDS Epidemic Update 2002*. [Online]. Available: http://www.unaids.org [accessed December 2002].

Ursin G, Spicer DV, Pike MC. 1994. Contraception and cancer prevention. *Adv Contracept Deliv Syst* 10(3-4):369–386.

Varila E, Wahlstrom T, Rauramo I. 2001. A 5-year follow-up study on the use of a levonorgestrel intrauterine system in women receiving hormone replacement therapy. *Fertil Steril* 76(5):969–973.

Wildemeersch D, Batar I, Webb A, Gbolade BA, Delbarge W, Temmerman M, Dhont M, Guillebaud J. 1999. GyneFIX: the frameless intrauterine contraceptive implant—an update for interval, emergency and postabortal contraception. *Br J Fam Plann* 24(4):149–159.

Wilson TE, Koenig L, Ickovics J, Walter E, Suss A, Fernandez MI. 2003. Contraception use, family planning, and unprotected sex: few differences among HIV-infected and uninfected postpartum women in four US states. *J Acquir Immune Defic Syndr* 33(5):608–613.

World Health Organization (WHO). 1992. *Oral Contraceptives and Neoplasia*. WHO Technical Report Series No. 817. Geneva, Switzerland: WHO. Pp. 1–46.

World Health Organization (WHO). 1998. *Cardiovascular Disease and Steroid Hormone Contraception*. World Health Organization Technical Report Series No. 877. Geneva, Switzerland: WHO.

World Health Organization Department of Reproductive Health and Research. 2000. *Annual Technical Report*. [Online]. Available: http://www.who.int/reproductive-health/pcc2001/Documents/mip%20exsum.pdf [accessed August 2003].

Xiao X, Yimin C, Shixiu G. 1999. Study into the reasons for unintended pregnancy. *Chinese Journal of Planned Parenthood Research* 7(10):446–448.

Zotti ME, Siegel E. 1995. Preventing unplanned pregnancies among married couples: are services for only the wife sufficient? *Res Nurs Health* 18(2):133–142.

5

Capitalizing on Recent Scientific Advances

Scientific advances are exciting in their own right for their contribution to the world of knowledge, but only if those advances can be transformed into practical applications will they have an impact on people's daily lives. Contraception is no exception; discoveries in the laboratory need to be translated into safe and effective devices and drugs that can be used by the people who need them.

There are, however, many barriers to this translational process. For example, adequate funding, researchers with expertise in the field, and collaboration among disciplines are all necessary for research to advance toward real applications. The regulatory process can also have an impact on the ability of research to advance to usable products.

The committee examined a number of pivotal issues that could influence the ease and speed with which its recommendations could be implemented and substantive progress made in the development and introduction of new and improved contraceptives.

ELEMENTS REQUIRED FOR PROGRESS IN CONTRACEPTIVE RESEARCH AND DEVELOPMENT

The blueprint for contraceptive research and product development outlined in this report can be realized only if several key elements are in place, including financial resources wisely deployed, human capital, a research environment that encompasses multiple disciplines relevant to contraception, a framework for increasing effective collaboration among the interested parties in the public and private sectors both in the United

States and abroad, and a regulatory environment conducive to contraceptive development. Educational and advocacy efforts are also needed to raise awareness about the benefits of family planning and the great need for new and improved contraceptive methods, both in the United States and abroad. All of these elements are closely interconnected; none alone can ensure success. Consequently, there is a need to address all of the issues simultaneously.

Adequate Funding

Development of a contraceptive product is expensive and time-consuming. The cost of developing a drug, from target discovery to approval, is $403 million to $802 million (Frank, 2003). Without the active engagement of large pharmaceutical companies, this amount of money is prohibitive.

The long-term funding horizon for contraceptive research is also a hurdle, as the timeline for drug development averages 10 to 14 years. Consequently, investments made in research for contraceptive development need to be long term if the goal is to see discoveries through to application and to ensure that a pipeline of emerging modalities will continue to meet changing needs. Sporadic funding may allow dabbling, but a sustained commitment is needed to see fundamental science translated into application. To accomplish the research and development goals and make the most of the targeted opportunities identified in this report, there must be sufficient and sustained financial support.

Where will the money come from? Historically, contraceptive research and development in the United States have been funded by the National Institutes of Health (NIH), other federal programs, foundations, venture capital, and industry. The levels of investment by the pharmaceutical industry vary, and the amounts invested by the various companies are generally not disclosed. However, the number of pharmaceutical and biotechnology companies that have invested programs in contraceptive development is modest. The trend for contraceptive funding from most other sources has been stagnant or declining. Although benefiting from the recent overall doubling of the NIH budget in 2001 and 2002, from 1980 to 2000, funding for contraceptive research in the NIH branches primarily dealing with this area of science was essentially flat in terms of constant dollars (Figure 5.1). Several foundations that have been significant sponsors of biomedical research related to contraception in the past, including the Ford Foundation, the Rockefeller Foundation, and the Andrew W. Mellon Foundation, have redirected their resources to other areas. Funding for population activities from the U.S. Agency for International Development (USAID) has also been essentially flat for the last 5 years. The

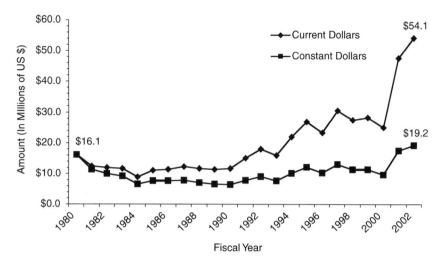

FIGURE 5.1 Consolidated Budget for the Contraceptive Development Branch, the Contraceptive and Reproductive Evaluation Branch, and the Contraception and Reproductive Health Branch of NICHD, 1980 to 2002. Note that the increased budgets for fiscal years 2001 and 2002 also include significant increases in reproductive health research in addition to contraceptive research, and that other NIH institutes also support some contraceptive research activities.
SOURCE: Contraception and Reproductive Health Branch, 2004.

following sections describe the rationale for support from these sources, as well as strategies to enhance research progress with the funds that become available.

A Rationale for Increased Federal Support

The United States has the largest biomedical research enterprise in the world, and the strongest pharmaceutical industry. Its research and product development capabilities, if directed toward contraception, could dramatically alter the future of fertility regulation. The development of new contraceptives benefits not only men and women in the United States but also men, women, and families worldwide. Responding to the national unmet needs for contraception is a matter of American self-interest, and deploying the nation's intellectual and technical resources to address the problem of fertility control and family planning worldwide helps fulfill the humanitarian responsibility of the United States. Success in this area can provide indirect benefits to the United States through increased political and economic stability and through better stewardship of the environment, leading to improved quality of life globally (Institute of

Medicine, 1997). Contraception is a very cost-effective means of improving quality of life and reproductive health through prevention (Shepard et al., 2003). The benefits of improving contraceptive methods and accessibility of contraception have been well documented (see Chapter 1). The facts about reduced morbidity and mortality and the benefits of positioning families and women physically, socially, and economically to embark on future pregnancies are, in the committee's opinion, more compelling than the rhetoric that has frequently surrounded debate regarding the commitment of federal dollars to family planning-related activities. Dissemination of these facts to legislators and the public would provide a powerful case for increased federal support. This rationale should be equally compelling to foundations and angel investors[1] who are committed to making a measurable difference in the quality of people's lives around the world. Importantly, congressional action can augment contraceptive research in ways other than simply appropriating more funds for contraceptive research and development (for example, by creating incentives for increased activity in industry).

Incentives to the Pharmaceutical Industry

The commitment of industry is critical for advances in contraceptive research and product development. To encourage continued and expanded efforts in this area, the committee considered several possible strategies, including patent life extension and favored tax status, for research and product development devoted to contraceptives. Contraceptives fall into a class of public health drugs and devices that might arguably deserve special recognition by the U.S. Congress through legislation similar to the Best Pharmaceuticals for Children Act (U.S. Congress, 2001) or the Orphan Drug Act (Food and Drug Administration, 1983). As noted in the 1996 Institute of Medicine (IOM) report, protection for product liability is also of considerable importance (Institute of Medicine, 1996). Indeed, some contraceptive methods (e.g., the Norplant implant and the Copper-7 intrauterine device [IUD]) that were approved by FDA as safe and effective were withdrawn from the U.S. market as a result of tort litigation (Institute of Medicine, 1998; Society for the Advancement of Women's Health Research, 1995). Indemnification for public health pharmaceuticals such as vaccines exists, and it is not unreasonable to extend the same arguments surrounding the legislation for vaccines to contraceptive drugs and

---

[1]Individuals who invest in a start-up company or in product development, often at a very early stage of development.

devices as important and necessary preventive agents (McCauley et al., 2002).

A Strategy for Wise Use of Funds

Contraceptive research is already using cutting-edge technology for novel target identification. Scientific opportunities abound, but careful target selection is mandatory given the cost of translating a target into a product. In the field of contraceptive research, a major bottleneck is the lack of funds for translational research and development, in which a target identified in the basic science stage undergoes testing for proof of concept and then on to product development. Thus, focusing investments on the most promising targets will maximize progress.

The challenge of funding the development of a contraceptive is magnified by the demand for multiple contraceptive modalities to meet the needs of both women and men, issues of appropriateness and acceptability for different populations, the cost of the product, and the complexity of product introduction and monitoring. The spectrum of biomedical research is displayed in Figure 5.2 as a linear process from earliest discovery to clinical application. Contraceptive research transcends this linear array, requiring a constant interaction among the disciplines to ensure that the end product is both effective and acceptable. While all of these elements may be important for the development of many therapeutic agents, the feedback loops for contraceptive development are far more complex. For example, contraception entails prevention rather than treatment, it is used by healthy people, and it may be continued over a 30-year period, so the tolerance of undesirable side effects is very low. In addition, the criteria used to measure the efficacy of pregnancy prevention are different from those used to determine the efficacy of a drug used to treat a disease. Moreover, reproduction is an intensely personal issue that is affected by cultural and social mores, so various methods will not be universally accepted. These issues raise the important question of whether current research and development structures are suitable for these efforts.

A structure or process for reaching the "go–no go" decisions that incorporates the wisdom of multiple disciplines and parties with diverse interests is needed in the public sector. There is no central coordinating body or interagency working group on the specific topic of contraception. Collaboration occurs through the major governmental, nongovernmental, and not-for-profit participants in contraceptive research and development, such as USAID, the National Institute of Child Health and Human Development (NICHD), the Centers for Disease Control and Prevention (CDC), the World Health Organization (WHO), Family Health International (FHI), the Population Council, and CONRAD, which col-

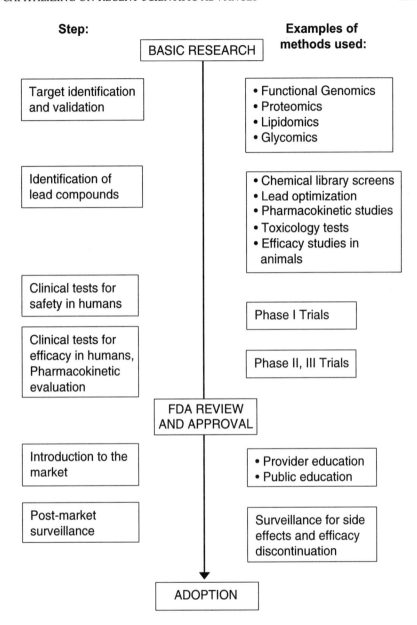

FIGURE 5.2 The spectrum of biomedical research displayed as a linear process from earliest discovery to clinical application.

laborate on an ad hoc basis to pursue various leads of mutual interest. In addition, the advisory committee meetings for Consortium for Industrial Collaboration in Contraceptive Research (CICCR)–CONRAD (CONRAD is the parent organization of CICCR), FHI, and the Population Council's International Committee for Contraception Research (ICCR) provide an ongoing forum for interchange of the most current scientific information, although this is more or less restricted to U.S.-based activities. NICHD is usually represented at these advisory committee meetings, but reproductive biology researchers rarely attend.

In contrast, three initiatives that provide information, collaboration, and support have been established in the related field of microbicide development. These collaborative arrangements illustrate constructive approaches to needs that still exist in contraceptive research.

The International Working Group on Microbicides was established in 1993 to attempt to harmonize activities in the field of microbicides, including recommendations about new regulatory issues arising from the development of vaginal microbicides and the standardization of colposcopy as a method for assessing vaginal irritation caused by microbicides (United Nations Population Fund, 2003). This standardization has been encapsulated in a colposcopy manual (CONRAD/WHO, 2002). This group meets on an ad hoc basis. Owing to the interest of a network of microbicide investigators, a series of international meetings on microbicides was organized and started in 2000, with meetings subsequently held every two years. These meetings have provided a forum for the exchange of current knowledge in research and development in microbicides and for networking researchers. The organizing committee has changed over the years, but it comprises a select number of individuals representing organizations active in the field who continue from one meeting to the next.

The Alliance for Microbicide Development,[2] established in 1998, acts as a clearinghouse for all new information on microbicides and keeps an up-to-date database showing the progress of all current lead compounds through the research and development pipeline. One level of the database is open to all and contains only information that is in the public domain or that is not proprietary. The second level contains proprietary information about the various lead compounds and is open only to developers and their collaborators and to potential funders. This organization captures all current relevant information and circulates it to a wide list of interested parties by e-mail on a weekly basis.

A third group, the International Partnership for Microbicides, was established in 2002 as a result of a study supported by the Rockefeller

---

[2]See http://www.microbicide.org/ (accessed August 2003).

Foundation to act as a coordinating body and central repository of funds for accelerating progress in the microbicide field (International Partnership for Microbicides, 2002) and has received generous support from the Bill and Melinda Gates Foundation and several other donors. Most current developers of microbicides are small biotechnology companies, not-for-profit organizations, and academic institutions with limited funding. Partnership with the International Partnership for Microbicides could potentially help these organizations identify and overcome gaps in research and development, access, and public awareness. The mode of operation of the International Partnership for Microbicides is still developing, so it is too early to assess its contribution to the field. One challenge that the organization faces is to avoid duplication of other efforts in the field.

The initiatives in the field of microbicides described above were instructional to the committee as it explored the merits of establishing similar resources to connect the different disciplines involved in contraceptive research and to provide investigators in contraceptive research those things that the International Working Group on Microbicides provides investigators in microbicide research. The current situation in contraceptive research is not satisfactory. For instance, at the recent annual meetings of all the major U.S. scientific societies that have reproductive biology as a major focus, for example, the Society for the Study of Reproduction,[3] the Society for Gynecologic Investigation,[4] and the American Society for Reproductive Medicine,[5] either very few or no papers dealt with basic or translational research in contraception. Whether this was a result of a lack of scientific interest, a lack of funding, or a lack of knowledge about the advances and needs in the field is not clear.

On an international level, regular meetings dealing with reproductive health already occur. For example, meetings of the World Congress of Gynecology and Obstetrics, the World Congress of Fertility and Sterility,[6] the World Congress on Human Reproduction,[7] and the Society for Advancement of Reproductive Care, all of which are held every 3 years,

---

[3]Society for the Study of Reproduction. 2003. *Society for the Study of Reproduction Home Page*. [Online]. Available: http://www.ssr.org/ (accessed August 2003).
[4]The Society for Gynecologic Investigation. *The Society for Gynecologic Investigation Home Page*. 2003. [Online]. Available: http://sgionline.org/ (accessed August 2003).
[5]The American Society for Reproductive Medicine. 2003. *The American Society for Reproductive Medicine Home*. [Online]. Available: http://www.infertilityprofessionals.com/clinical/asrm.html (accessed August 2003).
[6]International Federation of Fertility Societies. 2003. *IFFS 18th World Congress on Fertility and Sterility*. [Online]. Available: http://www.iffs2004.com/ (accessed August 2003).
[7]International Academy of Human Reproduction. 2003. *12th World Congress*. [Online]. Available: http://www.humanrep2005.org/academy.htm#2 (accessed August 2003).

are helpful; but given the long interval between such international congresses, presentations tend not to be a good source of current information. An information-gathering and exchange mechanism in the contraceptive research field would be of value. Such an organization, modeled after the Alliance for Microbicide Development, could be called the Alliance for Contraceptive Development. This endeavor would be worthy of investment and support.

In addition, because research programs tend to focus on their own interests, a case can be made for the establishment of a body of experts to review progress in the field at regular intervals and to make recommendations for future directions. Each research program has its own mandate and operating procedures, so it might be difficult for researchers to respond to a central oversight committee on contraceptive research and development as well as to their funders. Lessons learned from WHO task forces (Butler, 1993) will be informative. For example, the history of the Task Force on Male Contraception, recently reviewed by Geoffrey Waites (2003), reveals deficiencies that retarded the development of products and clinical trials. However, one mechanism that has been used in other fields and by individual programs in contraceptive research (including CONRAD, and Family Health International, and the Population Council) has been external evaluation boards, which not only provide guidance for the future but also reassure the funders that the progress in the field of contraceptives as a whole is on track and of high quality. Examples of this type of body include the Recombinant DNA Advisory Committee (Recombinant DNA Advisory Committee, 2000), but no similar body exists in the field of contraceptive development. Such an evaluation board could provide a road map that would be implemented in whole or in part, depending on the amount of funding provided. Given that international consortia are often influenced by the specific agendas of particular nations, the focus of any steering organization should strictly be on science and prototype product development, with individual nations or regions left to modify methods for their own unique needs.

Another strategy for improving dialogue among the various stakeholders in a rapidly changing scientific field is a roundtable or forum. That approach has been successfully used in other areas of biomedical research, such as microbial threats and clinical research.[8] A forum in contraception could provide a convening mechanism for interested parties from the academic, industrial, consumer, philanthropic, international

---

[8]See http://www.iom.edu/project.asp?id=3924 and http://www.iom.edu/project.asp?id=4881 (accessed September 2003).

health, medicine, public health, nursing, and federal research and regulatory perspectives to meet and discuss sensitive and difficult issues of mutual interest in a neutral setting. The purpose would be to foster dialogue and discussion across sectors and institutions and to illuminate but not necessarily resolve issues. The roundtable membership would determine the specific topics to discuss at its meetings, by weighing the interests of all parties and selecting issues of broad concern.

Depending on the topics and the intended audience, the forum might conduct public workshops, regional meetings, and other small workshops. Each of these would be designed to inform the discussion of issues related to contraceptive research and development but would not provide advice or recommendations. However, the forum could also identify and suggest topics for separate, independent study by other groups.

The creation of an Alliance for Contraceptive Development and a Contraception Roundtable are two strategies for promoting further collaboration between the public and the private sectors; working through decisions on priorities; and evaluating on an ongoing basis the status of research, development, and product introduction.

Staffing and Training

Human Capital

A cadre of scientists and physicians dedicated to contraceptive development is needed to implement the contraceptive research agenda. Although no one tracks data on investigator training or the workforce in the specific field of contraception, the committee believes that there is a paucity of such individuals in academe, that those who are active are aging, and that prospects for new blood seem bleak. For example, few if any scientific papers on contraception are presented at national meetings devoted to research on reproduction. This situation may be a reflection of the perceived lack of importance of the problem, the applied nature of contraceptive development research, the long time frame needed to bring the work to completion, and the meager funding available. A major challenge is to identify, attract, train, and support the career development of individuals who have an appreciation for the multidisciplinary issues surrounding fertility regulation. Increasing the pool of basic, translational, clinical, and social science investigators, and project managers dedicated to contraceptive research and development, will require a significant departure from the current ways in which investigators are trained as well as a specialized environment; but these changes are necessary for the research and development needed in the field of contraception.

The importance of contraceptive development as a national and global public health challenge must be appreciated if talented investigators are to be attracted to the field. To encourage young investigators, there must also be the promise of a future in such a career—primarily, adequate opportunities to obtain research funding. The academic community itself must also appreciate the unique features of contraceptive development research so that those who pursue activities that may be viewed as being outside the traditional path (i.e., applied research or team-based research) are not penalized. This will require a concerted effort to inform and support an academic environment conducive to encouraging investigators to pursue a career in contraceptive research.

Financial incentives are also strong magnets. Examples include employment opportunities as well as rewards for entering into and continuing in the field. The NIH Loan Repayment Program[9] is an excellent example of a financial incentive that could have a significant influence on career choice (Box 5.1). The committee hopes that this program will continue in the future and that it will place a special emphasis on individuals pursuing careers in contraceptive research. In addition, enhanced salary opportunities for individuals entering into the contraceptive research field would be beneficial. Given the long period of time required to make substantive contributions that lead to development of new products, the committee recognizes the need for support for junior or midlevel faculty and favors the establishment of endowed support to attract the most capable midlevel scientists in the field. Nongovernmental sources of funding to establish such endowments, such as from foundations, industry, or even committed individuals, are all appropriate for fostering work in contraceptive research. Finally, a significant prize for major achievements in contraceptive research and development could raise the visibility of the field in the eyes of the research community, the government, and the population at large.

Attracting and retaining physician-investigators represents another significant challenge, given the declining numbers of clinician-scientists. The demand for clinical productivity in academic medical centers detracts from research activities and promotes a harsh division between service and scholarship. In the absence of a system that welcomes and supports major emphasis on research, there will be continuing attrition in the ranks of physician-investigators. Mechanisms need to be put into place to secure support for physician-scientists in the junior and midcareer years, perhaps in the form of renewable career development awards or endowed faculty positions. Additionally, the shortage of medical expertise in critical disciplines such as andrology may impede progress in male contraception.

---

[9]See http://www.lrp.nih.gov/about/extramural/CIR/ (accessed August 2003).

**BOX 5.1
The NIH Loan Repayment Program**

NIH Loan Repayment Programs (LRP) offer repayment of educational loan debt of up to $35,000 per year for health professionals pursuing careers in contraception and infertility research (CIR-LRP), pediatric research, health disparities research, and clinical research (for individuals from disadvantaged backgrounds).

CIR-LRP provides for the repayment of the educational loan debts of qualified health professionals (including graduate students) who agree to commit to a period of obligated service of not less than two years conducting research on contraception or infertility at a National Institute of Child Health and Human Development (NICHD) intramural laboratory or at an eligible, approved NICHD-supported extramural site. CIR-LRP pays up to $35,000 of the principal and interest of such individuals' educational loans for each year of obligated service. Since 1997, 46 individuals have participated in CIR-LRP. Currently there are 16 active participants in CIR-LRP, which is 2 percent of the total number of participants (730). Of the participants in CIR-LRP, approximately 17 percent (8 of 46) have been involved in contraceptive research, with the rest of the participants focusing on infertility. This may be because of the activities of the eligible sites, most of which focus on infertility research.

Research on contraceptive topics being conducted through CIR-LRP includes contraceptive efficacy and safety, capacitation as a target for male contraception, and oocyte development.

SOURCE: Joan C. Davis, director, Contraception & Infertility Loan Repayment Program, Reproductive Sciences Branch, NICHD (http://www.lrp.nih.gov/about/ and http://www.lrp.nih.gov/about/extramural/CIR/) [accessed August 2003].

Some learned societies focus on contraception and population research, as well as offer postdoctoral training programs, such as those sponsored by the Buffett Foundation to provide opportunities for research and further training in the field of contraception. However, the United States has no means to recognize health care providers whose training gives them special competence in the specific area of contraception and related problems of reproductive health (e.g., sexually transmitted diseases). In contrast, in the early 1980s, the Royal College of Obstetricians and Gynaecologists of the United Kingdom developed subspecializations in five fields related to gynecology,[10] including one that was renamed Sexual and Reproductive Health in 2001. The subspecialists are defined as "obstetricians and gynecologists who, having undertaken appropriate additional higher training, are recognized to have special expertise in the relevant field. This higher degree of specialization indicates intensive training, experience and expertise." The program includes a theoretical aspect that focuses on understanding of sexual and reproductive health, contraceptive methods and mechanisms, and management and administration issues. It also includes a clinical aspect with training in contraception; unplanned pregnancy management, including termination; screening for diseases of the reproductive tract; care of women during menopause; psychosexual problems; prepregnancy counseling; and genitourinary medicine. Finally, there is a focus on applications for leading and managing a community-based service. A similar training program is being developed in France and is expected to begin in 2004.

Although formal recognition of a similar type might not be easily achieved in the United States or even enthusiastically received by the specialty and subspecialty organizations, the committee believes that it would be useful for existing training programs to work collaboratively to ensure that their trainees are recognized as experts through either learned societies or organizations. The American Society for Reproductive Medicine's Contraception Special Interest Group could be one such vehicle. Granting an appropriate degree (e.g., a master's degree) for trainees who complete a rigorous program could also be a mechanism to increase visibility and raise the stature of contraceptive research and practice among medical practitioners and researchers. This is, in fact, a component of some programs in the United States. The two-year Fellowship in Family Planning,[11] like the program in the United Kingdom, focuses on both clinical care and clinical research. Training in clinical care includes all methods of family planning currently available and under investigation, including the Norplant implant and IUDs; gynecologic surgery, including anesthesia and pain control; treatment of complications and hysterectomy; and all methods of pregnancy termination. The research training includes study design, grant writing, and statistical analysis; and it offers opportunities and guidance for research studies. This program differs from the one in the United Kingdom in that it does not grant any official

---

[10]Royal College of Obstetricians and Gynaecologists Faculty of Family Planning and Reproductive Health Syllabus for Subspecialisation in Sexual and Reproductive Health: SRH.1—Syllabus. The Faculty of Family Planning & Reproductive Health Care, May 2003.

[11]Fellowship in Family Planning, http://familyplanningfellowship.org/ (accessed September 2003). Also, personal communication with Mitchell Creinin, University of Pittsburgh School of Medicine, 1 of the 12 fellowship directors.

degrees or provide any certification. However, the need for increased training in this area is slowly being recognized; recent advertisements for specialists trained through fellowships in this area show an increased demand for such training. The program provides extensive training in contraception, which is often not provided in medical school, and aims for its graduates to be resources for training other residents and students. There are currently 12 fellowship positions each year nationwide, 10 in obstetrics-gynecology and 2 in family practice.

The Research and Training Environment

Development of contraceptives requires familiarity with many other fields and not just competence in contraception. Many excellent research programs with strengths in reproductive biology or clinical research exist in the United States and abroad. Few, however, have the necessary breadth—spanning basic science, translational and clinical research, social science and demographics, as well as established relationships with industry—to facilitate product development. Centers currently involved in contraceptive research should be encouraged to address this deficit and weave the social and demographic sciences into the process of contraceptive research and development.

The multidisciplinary nature of contraceptive development research requires a team approach, as opposed to the traditional investigator-initiated research approach prevalent in U.S. academic institutions. This type of team-based approach with an application goal is the norm in industry, where individuals are rewarded for their contributions to successful teams. Fundamental changes in the process by which science is conducted are needed to facilitate translational research and product development. A change in the culture of the research enterprise is not unheard of, but such a change may need to be sold to academe so that individual participants are not penalized in terms of career advancement, such as delays in promotion or tenure.

The multidisciplinary nature of contraceptive development could also benefit from the advent of the "large-scale science" approach that has emerged during the past decade as a new paradigm in biomedical research (Institute of Medicine, 2003). For example, a large-scale collaborative approach was used in the Human Genome Project and in the efforts to develop new therapies for HIV/AIDS.[12] This has led to a wealth of new

---

[12]The approach used for the rapid development of new drugs for HIV infection and AIDS included federally supported networks for conducting clinical trials, which were set up in addition to the huge influx of grant dollars. There were also collaborative efforts with industry, e.g., the AIDS Drug Development Task Force convened by the U.S. Department of Health and Human Services.

information based on collaborative arrangements previously not the norm in biomedical research. The lessons learned from multidisciplinary or team-based science can be applied to contraceptive development. One possible model through which diverse resources from the academic community could be marshaled is the NICHD cooperative agreement programs, which are beginning to forge multi-institutional research teams that focus on specific areas of reproductive science. Linking this consortium with industry would further facilitate contraceptive development.

Team-based science may benefit from being more international in scope as well. A number of talented and productive investigators outside of the United States have excellent resources for clinical investigation, but there are barriers to working with them. Only a small pool of U.S. investigators has experience in international research. Furthermore, international research collaborations can be derailed by differences in regulatory requirements for human subjects' protection, informed consent, and privacy.

The provision of supplemental funding to U.S. investigators for international collaborations and team science is one mechanism that could be used to encourage these activities and that could augment not only research but also research training. Examples of this approach that are directly relevant to contraceptive research include the Mellon Foundation's twinning program (Makinson and Harper, 1999),[13] which had limited funds to foster these interactions but which will soon cease.[14] Other international research programs include the Fogarty International Research Collaboration Awards (Fogarty International Center/National Institute of Environmental Health Sciences, 2002),[15] which target interactions between a funded U.S. investigator and foreign collaborator, and the Indo-U.S. Joint Working Group in Contraception and Reproductive Health.[16] These awards are also modest in size and, in the case of the U.S.-Indo Joint Working Group, limited in time.

---

[13]See http://www.reproline.jhu.edu/english/1fp/1advances/conrad.htm (accessed September 2003).

[14]See http://www.mellon.org/programs/population/population.htm (accessed September 2003).

[15]See http://grants.nih.gov/grants/guide/pa-files/PA-02-057.html (accessed August 2003).

[16]See http://grants1.nih.gov/grants/guide/notice-files/NOT-HD-03-009.html (accessed August 2003).

Increasing Collaboration

Collaboration Among Disciplines

In addition to collaboration among researchers across physical borders, research must cross disciplines as well throughout contraceptive development stages to improve the speed and success of the introduction of new contraceptive methods. The process of bringing contraceptive methods from the point of discovery through the development, testing, and introduction of the method demands input from experts from many disciplines, including but not limited to biologists, chemists, physical scientists, engineers, regulatory specialists, social scientists, and clinicians. Input across disciplines throughout development stages is essential to facilitate successful product development and introduction. Cross-collaboration may be especially difficult when contraceptive discovery and development take place in the public sector or among individual researchers outside the infrastructure of large pharmaceutical companies, which are organized to take product development through all the required stages.

Collaboration can potentially be hindered by competition among the various organizations in a particular research field, so it would be worthwhile to identify and support mechanisms that would facilitate and increase opportunities for such collaboration in contraceptive research both within the public sector and between public and private entities. These might include meetings focused on contraceptive approaches or on stages of method development sponsored by impartial groups such as NIH, IOM, WHO, the Population Council, CONRAD, and CICCR; funding for the early involvement of experts from fields that will be needed during method development; or funders' encouragement of cross-collaboration.

Public–Private Partnerships

The concept of establishing public–private partnerships (PPPs) to achieving progress in global health is well accepted. Significant examples include the International AIDS Vaccine Initiative and Global Alliance for TB (Tuberculosis) Drug Development. A recent publication from the Initiative on Public–Private Partnerships for Health has attempted to value industry contributions to PPPs (Kettler et al., 2003). Ten such PPP deals were examined. The authors concluded that large multinational corporations express reservations about working on diseases targeted by the PPPs such as malaria, tuberculosis, and HIV/AIDS. They noted four main concerns: unsolved access problems, negative public relations, unresolved intellectual property rights issues, and difficult scientific hurdles. All of these concerns apply to contraceptive research and development as well but are magnified and make this area even less appealing to large pharmaceutical companies. However, a productive relationship between industry and the public sector is essential for success in translating basic research findings to the clinical setting (Schwartz and Vilquin, 2003).

In the 1996 IOM report on contraceptive research and development, the committee commented that with a few notable exceptions, industry, broadly defined, has not found the potential rewards from the development of new contraceptive methods to be persuasive, given the greater chance of success and higher financial rewards in other areas of therapeutic intervention such as oncology. Contraception, which by definition involves prevention rather than cure, carries the added safety risks inherent in treating healthy people. That report also noted that "the contemporary pharmaceutical industry is a sequence of 'virtual partnerships' and contract research arrangements at different" stages of the research and development process (p. 19). The willingness of small companies to become engaged in PPPs was also noted favorably, but with the obvious caveats that they had only limited funding and that the time to drug approval is long.

An early example of a PPP was created for the development of the Copper T IUD through a collaboration between the Population Council and FEI Products in the early 1980s and the subsequent alliance with pharmaceutical marketers to introduce the product. The Copper T IUD, which has been available since 1984, has become the most widely used long-acting, reversible contraceptive in the world and provides 10 years of contraceptive efficacy for millions of women around the world (Sivin et al., 1994).

Major benefits of the PPP concept are not only to attract industry into a particular area but also to keep it interested and active in that area. This was the basis for the establishment of CICCR (Consortium for Industrial Collaboration in Contraceptive Research, 2000). In the 1996 IOM report, the committee expressed its belief that the CICCR initiative was a creative and potentially high-payoff mechanism for sponsor investment. CICCR's feasibility grants support innovative high-risk research with seed money to test a concept or obtain preliminary results on research that would make a project more attractive to an industrial partner. CICCR's matching funds program fosters collaboration between research institutions and pharmaceutical companies. It provides funds to investigators at not-for-profit institutions that have projects of interest to industry. CICCR was established at CONRAD in 1995 (CONRAD, 2001) with funding from a philanthropic foundation in the hope that the model would attract other donors. Since CONRAD was already receiving funding from USAID, CDC, and

NICHD, additional funds could leverage efforts in contraceptive research. CICCR had three priority areas of contraceptive research: male methods, monthly methods for women, and vaginal methods that would be both contraceptive and prevent against sexually transmitted infections (STIs), including HIV infection. These areas are the same as those cited in the first recommendation of the 1996 IOM report. This model proved attractive to five other foundations and the United Nations Population Fund, which became donors at various times. Some, but not all, continue to participate. Additional funding specifically earmarked for the development of vaginal preparations to prevent HIV infection and other STIs permitted the establishment of a sister project, the Global Microbicide Project (Global Microbicide Project, 2000). Progress toward the stated objectives of CICCR has been assessed by external review committees of the program as a whole as well as the individual program areas and is documented in the CICCR–Global Microbicide Project 2001–2002 Biennial Report, *Addressing Reproductive Health Needs* (CICCR (Consortium for Industrial Collaboration in Contraceptive Research), 2003).

In addition to CICCR, several other partnerships relevant to contraceptive development have been established since 1996. The Rockefeller Foundation partnered in a one-time 5-year agreement with Schering AG to fund basic research on the epididymis with the purpose of identifying new targets for male contraception. This project, known as Application of Molecular Pharmacology for Post-Testicular Activity (AMPPA) (CICCR, 2003), ran from 1998 to 2002 and was so successful that Schering AG indicated its willingness to continue, provided that another partner could be found as a successor to the Rockefeller Foundation. CICCR has now entered into a new agreement with Schering AG called Application of Molecular Pharmacology for Post-Meiotic Activity (AMPPA-2), which commenced in 2003 for an initial period of only 3 years because of limits of assured future funding. During this same time period, the Population Council licensed its testosterone-like hormone MENT (7-α-methyl-19-nortestosterone) to Schering AG for development and use in male hormone replacement and contraception. The partnership between the Population Council and Schering AG continues, and the two organizations are jointly guiding the development and testing of various forms of delivery for this product with strong potential for widespread use.

The Rockefeller Foundation also made a one-time 5-year grant to WHO (Butler, 1993; World Health Organization, 2000) for support of the Initiative on Implantation, since apart from support for basic reproductive research by NICHD and work supported by CICCR in its Monthly Methods for Women program, no other funding was available for such targeted research on postfertilization methods. Indeed, Recommendation 5 of the 1996 IOM report stressed that "research and development of anti-implantation methods be pursued as a response to major health need and to evidence of demand" (p. 15). The committee recognized that at the early stages, industrial involvement might be limited because of the controversial nature of such research. Nevertheless, this was believed to be a priority area for support from funders for whom the controversy was not constraining. This partnership ran from 1999 to 2003.

Since 2000, the investigators supported by CICCR and the WHO–Rockefeller Foundation initiative have met about once a year to exchange information and establish research collaborations. These meetings have been highly valued by the participants, and confidential reports prepared jointly by grantees and external advisers have been highly complimentary of the progress achieved. The most recent meeting of the two programs in Bellagio, Italy, in 2003 (World Health Organization, 2003) brought together investigators who had studied the most promising biological targets and representatives of industry with the specific intention of attracting support for further development. Although the specifics of the private discussions are unknown, it appears that at least some matches for collaboration were made. There is also the possibility of establishing a program similar to AMPPA-2, but for research on female contraception. Once again, however, continuance of a valuable initiative may lapse without the assistance of other funders.

Public–private partnerships have been instrumental in bringing several contraceptives to market, including the Norplant implant and the Plan B emergency contraceptive method. Work on the technology behind Norplant was begun by the Population Council in the 1960s and continued through 1990, when FDA approval was granted. A pharmaceutical company in Finland, Leiras Oy, developed the manufacturing procedures; and Wyeth Ayerst provided funding for introduction of the implant into the U.S. market, including the training of 27,000 clinicians in the techniques of implant insertion, removal, and appropriate counseling. Postmarketing surveillance and acceptability studies were undertaken in a wide range of countries with the involvement of the Population Council, WHO, FHI, and the Program for Appropriate Technologies in Health (Institute of Medicine, 1998).

In the case of Plan B, Women's Capital Corporation took responsibility for bringing to market the emergency contraceptive method long known to clinicians when the pharmaceutical industry would not because of litigation and public relations concerns. Oversight of clinical trials, data management and analysis, formulation development, registration, manufacturing, packaging, warehousing and distribution, market introduction, quality assurance, accounting, and sales of Plan B were all accomplished using a virtual organization staffed by three persons. Thus, a large bricks and mortar institution is not essential for all stages of product development. Recently, Barr Laboratories, Inc., one of the largest producers of generic oral contraceptives, signed a letter of intent to acquire Plan B from Women's Capital Corporation. This is an example of a partnership of angel investors, foundations, and WHO that transitioned to the pharmaceutical industry.

It should be noted, however, that for both the Norplant implant and Plan B, the concept and drugs were already established. The partnerships shepherded the methods through the clinical trials and regulatory hurdles. The stories might have been considerably different if the efforts had started from an early stage of target discovery and development of the methods. Such an undertaking would require expanded partnerships between the public and private sectors to translate promising lead compounds into clinically useful products (Schwartz and Vilquin, 2003).

The committee concludes that PPPs are an effective mechanism to advance research in reproductive health and contraception and that such initiatives have high payoffs for sponsors that invest in them. Combining the complementary strengths of the not-for-profit and for-profit sectors facilitates progress in the translation of lead compounds into products. However, PPPs do not need to focus only on a specific target molecule but can also be used for more basic research using the tools of modern technology to identify new targets, as shown by the AMPPA agreements, which were new types of collaborations. The success of CICCR during the last 8 years shows the sturdiness of the PPP mechanism and its ability to work in important, although controversial, areas, such as postfertilization methods of contraception. Thus, increased collaboration among public-sector agencies, industry, and other organizations active in the field would accelerate contraceptive development. The support of philanthropic foundations in this effort is to be commended, but new funders are needed, as programmatic changes have resulted in two of the largest funders to withdraw from this field. One potential mechanism for NIH to promote pub-lic- private cooperation is the Small Business Technology Transfer (STTR) program, which was developed to foster technology transfer and commercialization between small businesses and research institutions such as universities and other nonprofit organizations.

Increased Participation by Developing Countries

New contraceptives that may be developed from target molecules identified by the new approaches to basic science will be used in a wide variety of cultural and political settings in countries at various stages of economic development. Thus, the needs of consumers have to be kept firmly in mind during the development process. Institutions in developing countries can clearly play a role in advising on preferred routes of administration and in the development of the vehicles or systems. For example, work was being conducted at the National Institute of Pharmaceutical Education and Research in India on different formulations of microbicides[17] (Damu et al., 2000; Garg, 1998; Garg et al., 2003). Continued funding could nurture a valuable resource for the field.

Some developing countries have already contributed to contraceptive research and are continuing to work in this area. For example, Cyclofem, the combination of progestin and estrogen in an injectable format, was originally developed in Brazil in 1968 (Coutinho and de Souza, 1968), the first progestin-only oral contraceptive was developed in Latin America (Coutinho, 1993), and Gossypol was first tested as a male contraceptive in China in the 1970s (National Co-ordinating Group for Male Contraceptives, 1978).

Many countries, such as Brazil, Chile, China, India, and Mexico, also have flourishing pharmaceutical industries that make reproductive health products, some of which can already produce drugs of Good Manufacturing Practice quality. For instance, companies in India (such as Ranbaxy, Cipla, and Dr. Reddy's Laboratories Limited) make generic and other drugs for sale in a variety of countries, including the United States. The Population Council collaborated with Laboratorios Silesia S.A. in Chile in the development of a progesterone vaginal ring for use as a contraceptive by lactating women and has licensed this product to that company for marketing in Chile, advancing the availability of a product that is particularly well suited to local conditions and preferences (Diaz et al., 1985, 1997). Greater efforts could be made to encourage such companies to become partners in the development of new target molecules and translation to a product, especially since locally produced products may be more widely accepted in the country setting. For example, a Mexican company, Applicaciones Farmaceuticas, manufactured the monthly hormonal contraceptive Cyclofem and then supported its introduction in the local market until the FDA approved it for the U.S. market as Lunelle. Thus, if pharmaceutical companies in developed countries are unwilling to partner in the development of new contraceptives, partnering with the pharmaceutical industry in developing countries is a viable option.

Many institutions in developing countries have also been involved in clinical trials of contraceptives, including India, Brazil, Chile, the Dominican Republic, China, South Africa, Zimbabwe, Kenya, Nigeria, Botswana, Côte d'Ivoire, Thailand, and others. Institutions in many of these countries conduct research under Good Clinical Practice standards and are willing and able to undertake additional studies, provided that funding is

---

[17]See http://niper.nic.in/ (accessed August 2003).

available. The per patient costs in such settings are usually considerably less than those incurred in developed country settings. Studies locally conducted can also lead to faster regulatory approval in that country. Involvement of investigators and institutions in contraceptive product research and development in developing countries has been the established mode of operation in the Population Council's ICCR since its establishment in 1970. Over the years membership has included clinicians from Brazil, Chile, the Dominican Republic, and India. Further use and expansion of such resources are to be encouraged. However, funding will be required not only for institution building but also for ensuring that clinical trial sites meet Good Clinical Practice standards.

For many years WHO has had an institution-building component in reproductive health, including contraceptive research, and has sponsored many multicenter clinical trials of contraceptives in a variety of developing countries.[18] Many of these have been seminal. Examples include studies demonstrating that the use of testosterone alone can provide contraception in Asian males, although for universal application a combination regimen that includes an androgen and the addition of a progestin will likely be needed (Aribarg et al., 1996; Bebb et al., 1996; Handelsman et al., 1995; Lei et al., 1996; Sukcharoen et al., 1996; World Health Organization Task Force on Methods for the Regulation of Male Fertility, 1990). Funding for continued research in such areas has been declining, but this is a resource that should not to be overlooked. Donors to the WHO Reproductive Health Division are urged to continue to support these research activities, as the WHO imprimatur counts for much in many countries.

Since 1993, the Mellon Foundation has also provided funds for collaboration between centers of excellence in the United States and developing countries through a twinning program (Makinson and Harper, 1999). It was hoped that greater exposure to developing countries would convince U.S. investigators of the importance of scientific advances in contraceptives suitable for those settings. These funds were awarded on a competitive basis by CONRAD. An external evaluation of the impact of this twinning program in 1999 was very favorable. For programmatic reasons, the Mellon Foundation has decided to terminate the population program, which includes both the twinning program and the support for the U.S. Reproductive Biology Centers. No new awards will be made after

---

[18]See *WHO: Capacity Strengthening* at http://www.who.int/reproductive-health/strategic_approach/ (accessed August 2003). Also see the U.N. Development Program/U.N. Population Fund/WHO/World Bank Special Programme of Research, Development and Research Training in Human Reproduction (HRP) main page at http://www.who.int/reproductive-health/hrp/index.html (accessed August 2003).

December 2004, and activity must cease by December 2005. However, alternative funding sources could potentially continue the benefits of the Mellon Foundation-initiated twinning program.

The Fogarty International Center has supported a somewhat similar program that provides competitive research grants (Fogarty International Research Collaboration Awards) to foreign investigators who are working on a collaborative project with a U.S. investigator holding an active research project grant. The Global Health in Research Initiative provides reentry grants on a competitive basis to foreign scholars who have had postdoctoral training at NIH or at academic centers sponsored by Fogarty International Center training grants. These programs are current, and perhaps with additional funding they could expand their numbers of awards.

Various other initiatives that involve collaboration with centers of excellence also exist. For example, the Indo-U.S. Joint Working Group on Contraceptives and Reproductive Health Research supports collaborative research between Indian and U.S. investigators. Funds are provided by both NICHD and USAID on the U.S. side and the Department of Biotechnology and the Indian Council for Medical Research on the Indian side. Notably, individual programs active in the contraceptive research and development field, such as CONRAD (CICCR and the Global Microbicide Project), FHI, Program for Appropriate Technology in Health, the Population Council, and WHO, have very active programs that involve collaboration with institutions worldwide not just for clinical trials but also for preclinical activities and feasibility and proof-of-concept studies.

Improving Dialogue with Regulatory Bodies

Contraceptive development requires a regulatory process that is dynamic, meaning that it keeps abreast of changing science, changing needs, and changing opportunities for product development. Regulatory agencies have traditionally established review principles based on existing classes of drugs or delivery systems. The process is more awkward with novel agents or approaches, which are an expected outcome of the research agenda outlined in this report. Consequently, contraceptive researchers need to be proactive in their interactions with regulatory bodies to ensure that the timeline for drug or device approval is efficient and that the regulatory requirements are appropriate, while they must also ensure that the highest standards for drug manufacture, safety, and monitoring are met. Dialogue is central to this endeavor; what is needed is dialogue based on the concerns of both the regulatory agencies and the sponsors to ensure safe and effective contraceptive methods. The recent formulation of regulatory guidelines for male contraceptives by investigators is an excellent example of the proactive approach (Nieschlag et al.,

2002). However, guidelines must be considered fluid, requiring continuous reevaluation to avoid the creation of rigid and outdated guidance that may impede rather than facilitate contraceptive drug and device development. Consequently, it is important that a dialogue and format be established as soon as possible so that any guidelines promulgated serve all parties well. Recent statements regarding FDA's interest in working in partnership with industry to facilitate drug registration potentially signal a new era in industry–FDA relationships (Bowe and Griffith, 2003; Griffith and McClellan, 2003). The committee urges FDA to hold public hearings on the current status of contraceptive research and the relevance of current guidances to today's emerging technologies.

The unification of regulatory requirements and processes across countries is being developed by the International Conference on Harmonisation of Technical Requirements for Registration of Pharmaceuticals for Human Use (ICH, 2003). Unfortunately, this process has been protracted and reflects difficulties in achieving international consensus even on seemingly noncontroversial technical matters. Under the auspices of regulatory harmonization, the committee also endorses international exchanges for investigators in the field of contraception. These could include exchanges of laboratory techniques as well as ethical approaches for conducting the clinical trials necessary for the review and approval of new contraceptives.

RECOMMENDATIONS

The blueprint for contraceptive research and product development outlined in this report can be realized only if several key elements are in place, including financial resources and a system to judiciously deploy them, human capital, a research environment that encompasses multiple disciplines relevant to contraception, a framework for increasing effective collaboration among the interested parties in the public and private sectors both in the United States and abroad, and a regulatory environment conducive to contraceptive development.

Recommendation 10: Expand public–private partnerships that draw on the complementary strengths of the public-sector agencies, industry, foundations, consumer groups, and other organizations to expedite the translation of lead compounds into contraceptive products.

Public–private partnerships have significant track records in attracting and retaining industry interest in a particular scientific area, and such partnerships have proven to be one effective mechanism to advance research in reproductive health and contraception. The complementary strengths of the not-for-profit and for-profit sectors are necessary to ensure rapid progress in the translation of lead compounds to products, and such initiatives appear to have a high payoff for sponsors that invest in them. The support of philanthropic foundations in promoting this concept is commendable, and further collaboration between public and private organizations active in the field would be worthwhile.

Recommendation 11: Facilitate collaboration between organizations in developed and developing countries in contraceptive development, clinical testing, and understanding of the acceptability of methods.

Increased cooperation between organizations in developed and developing countries could also speed and enhance contraceptive research and development. Nongovernmental organizations, governmental public health agencies, universities, research institutions, medical research councils, and industry in developing countries can make valuable contributions to contraceptive development in a variety of ways. First, institutions in developing countries can clearly play a role in determining preferred routes of administration and in the development of the delivery vehicles or systems. Second, some developing countries have active research programs in contraception, including work on injectables in Brazil and male contraceptives in China. Third, a number of developing countries have flourishing pharmaceutical industries, some of which already meet Good Manufacturing Practice standards. Fourth, many institutions in developing countries are involved in clinical trials of contraceptives. The cost of clinical trials is generally lower in these countries, and enrollment targets are often achieved faster. Thus, involvement of these organizations in contraceptive development should be encouraged and supported.

This goal could be accomplished by drawing on centers of excellence worldwide, especially in developing countries, to incorporate knowledge of local needs and preferences into research on methods that will be acceptable to different cultures. Collaboration with pharmaceutical companies in developing countries would also facilitate the rapid development of new contraceptive agents. In addition, it would be beneficial to engage sites in developing countries with expertise in conducting basic and clinical research on new contraceptives, and where necessary, to assist these sites in meeting Good Clinical Practice standards.

Recommendation 12: Establish, support, and recognize new programs for training and career advancement in contraceptive research and clinical practice.

A cadre of scientists and physicians dedicated to contraceptive development is needed to implement the contraceptive research agenda. A major challenge is to identify, attract, train, and support the career development of young investigators in basic, translational, clinical, and social sciences who have an interest and appreciation for the multidisciplinary issues surrounding fertility regulation. More postdoctoral training oppor-tunities are needed, and trainees who complete a rigorous program should be recognized as experts through learned societies or organizations. To encourage young investigators, there must also be the promise of a career future, primarily adequate opportunities to win research funding. Given the long period of time required to make substantive contributions in this field leading to the development of new products, the committee recog-nizes the need for support for junior or midlevel faculty and favors the establishment of endowed support to attract the most capable midlevel scientists in the field. The academic community itself must also appreciate the unique features of contraceptive development research so that those who pursue activities that may be viewed as being outside the traditional path (i.e., applied research or team-based research) are not penalized.

Recommendation 13: Create organizations to promote communica-tion among the many parties interested in contraceptive research and to serve as a clearinghouse for information on contraceptive research.

Wise use of available funding is essential to maximize progress in the field of contraceptive research. The difficulty of narrowing down a large number of possible targets is compounded by the multiplicity of disci-plines involved in contraceptive development, the high cost of product development, and the complexity of product introduction and monitor-ing. No central coordinating body, information source, or interagency working group on the specific topic of contraception exists.

In the related field of microbicide development, in contrast, the Alli-ance for Microbicide Development[19] acts as a clearinghouse for all new information on microbicides and keeps an up-to-date database showing the progress of all current lead compounds in the research and develop-ment pipeline. The development of such an organization, modeled after the Alliance for Microbicide Development, for the broader field of contra-ception would be worthy of investment and support.

Such an entity could facilitate and expand communication via the Internet among scientists involved in basic research on reproductive biology and contraceptive research and development and could also develop mechanisms for scientists from multiple disciplines and locations to interact and to share information and resources for the development of contraceptives. Expanded use of the Internet could also provide resource

---

[19]See http://www.microbicide.org/ (accessed August 2003).

information to scientists regarding drug delivery efforts in other research areas, analysis of current delivery systems in the contraceptive field, and contact information for contract laboratories. An Alliance for Contraceptive Development could stimulate and maintain public awareness and support for contraceptive research and development as well by providing ongoing information through an Internet site reporting the progress of research activities.

Another strategy for improving dialogue among the various stakeholders in a rapidly changing scientific field is a roundtable or forum. This approach has successfully been used in other areas of biomedical research, such as microbial threats and clinical research. In contrast to an Alliance for Contraceptive Development, which would collect resource material and disseminate information, a Forum on Contraceptive Research and Development would provide a mechanism to facilitate integration of the activities of different stakeholders and to foster dialogue and discussion across sectors and institutions.

REFERENCES

Aribarg A, Sukcharoen N, Chanprasit Y, Ngeamvijawat J, Kriangsinyos R. 1996. Suppression of spermatogenesis by testosterone enanthate in Thai men. *J Med Assoc Thai* 79(10):624–629.

Bebb RA, Anawalt BD, Christensen RB, Paulsen CA, Bremner WJ, Matsumoto AM. 1996. Combined administration of levonorgestrel and testosterone induces more rapid and effective suppression of spermatogenesis than testosterone alone: a promising male contraceptive approach. *J Clin Endocrinol Metab* 81(2):757–762.

Bowe C, Griffith V. 2003, July 31. FDA to speed up drug approvals system. *The Financial Times*, p. 1.

Butler D. 1993. WHO widens focus of AIDS research. *Nature* 366(6453):293.

CONRAD. 2001. *Making Progress toward Better Reproductive Health for All.* [Online]. Available: http://www.conrad.org/conradbien0001.final.pdf [accessed August 2003].

CONRAD/WHO. 2002. *Manual for the Standardization of Colposcopy for the Evaluation of Vaginal Products. Update 2002.* Arlington, VA: CONRAD and the World Health Organization.

Consortium for Industrial Collaboration in Contraceptive Research. 2000. *Funding for a Partnership between the Pharmaceutical Industry and Not-for-Profit Research Institutions: An Investment in the Early Stages of Drug Development for the New Contraceptive Technology Revolution.* [Online]. Available: http://www.conrad.org/about_ciccr.html [accessed August 2003].

Consortium for Industrial Collaboration in Contraceptive Research. 2003. *Addressing Reproductive Health Needs.* [Online]. Available: http://www.conrad.org/2003Biennialfinal. pdf [accessed August 2003].

Contraception and Reproductive Health Branch, NICHD. 2004. *Report to the NACHHD Council.* [Online]. Available: http://www.nichd.nih.gov/publications/pubs/coun_crh.htm [accessed January 2004].

Coutinho EM. 1993. Latin America's contributions to contraceptive development. *Fertil Steril* 60(2):227–230.

Coutinho EM, de Souza JC. 1968. Contraception control by monthly injections of medroxyprogesterone suspension and a long-acting estrogen. *J Reprod Fertil* 15:209–214.

Damu U, Vermani K, Garg S, Waller DP, Zaneveld LJ. 2000. Development and evaluation of a bioadhesive vaginal film for EGB, a novel antimicrobial contraceptive agent. *Indian J Pharm Sci* 62:505.

Diaz S, Zepeda A, Maturana X, Reyes MV, Miranda P , Casado ME, Peralta O, Croxatto HB. 1985. Fertility Regulation in Nursing Women, VIII: Progesterone plasma levels and contraceptive efficacy of a progesterone-releasing vaginal ring. *Contraception* 32:603–622.

Diaz S, Zepeda A, Maturana X, Reyes MV, Miranda P , Casado ME, Peralta O, Croxatto HB. 1997. Fertility regulation in nursing women: contraceptive performance, duration of lactation, infant growth, and bleeding patterns during use of progesterone vaginal rings, progestin-only pills, Norplant implants, and Copper T 380-A intrauterine devices. *Contraception* 56:223–232.

Fogarty International Center/National Institute of Environmental Health Sciences. 2002. *Fogarty National Research Collaboration Award (FIRCA)*. [Online]. Available: http://grants.nih.gov/grants/guide/pa-files/PA-02-057.html [accessed August 2003].

Food and Drug Administration. 1983. *The Orphan Drug Act (as amended)*. [Online]. Available: http://www.fda.gov/orphan/oda.htm [accessed August 2003].

Frank RG. 2003. New estimates of drug development costs. *J Health Econ* 22(2):325–330.

Garg S. 1998. Vaginal microbicide. *Pharm Sci Technol Today* 1:369.

Garg S, Kandarapu R, Vermani K, Tambwekar KR, Garg A, Waller DP, Zaneveld LJ. 2003. Development pharmaceutics of microbicide formulations. I: Preformulation considerations and challenges. *AIDS Patient Care STDs* 17(1):17–32.

Global Microbicide Project. 2000. *Global Microbicide Project . . . Responding to an Urgent Need*. [Online]. Available: http://www.gmp.org/ [accessed August 2003].

Griffith V, McClellan M. 2003, July 31. McClellan seeks to trim the fat. Interview. The new head of the FDA wants better labeling of food and faster approval of delivery of drugs to the US market. *The Financial Times*, p. 10.

Handelsman DJ, Farley TM, Peregoudov A, Waites GM. 1995. Factors in nonuniform induction of azoospermia by testosterone enanthate in normal men. World Health Organization Task Force on Methods for the Regulation of Male Fertility. *Fertil Steril* 63(1):125–133.

Institute of Medicine. 1996. *Contraceptive Research and Development: Looking to the Future*. Harrison PF, Rosenfield A, eds. Washington, DC: National Academy Press.

Institute of Medicine. 1997. *America's Vital Interest in Global Health: Protecting Our People, Enhancing Our Economy, and Advancing Our International Interests*. Washington, DC: National Academy Press.

Institute of Medicine. 1998. *Contraceptive Research, Introduction, and Use: Lessons From Norplant*. Harrison PF, Rosenfield A, eds. Washington, DC: National Academy Press.

Institute of Medicine. 2003. *Large-Scale Biomedical Science: Exploring Strategies for Future Research*. Nass SJ, Stillman BW, eds. Washington, DC: The National Academies Press.

International Conference on Harmonisation (ICH). 2003. *Welcome to the Official Website for ICH*. [Online]. Available: http://www.ich.org/ [accessed August 2003].

International Partnership for Microbicides. 2002. *About IPM*. [Online]. Available: http://www.ipm-microbicides.org [accessed August 2003].

Kettler H, White K, Jordan S. 2003. *Valuing Industry Contributions to Public–Private Partnerships for Health Product Development*. Geneva, Switzerland: The Initiative on Public-Private Partnerships for Health, Global Forum for Health Research.

Lei ZW, Wu SC, Garceau RJ, Jiang S, Yang QZ, Wang WL, Vander Meulen TC. 1996. Effect of pretreatment counseling on discontinuation rates in Chinese women given depomedroxyprogesterone acetate for contraception. *Contraception* 53(6):357–361.

Makinson C, Harper MJ. 1999. Pushing the frontiers of science: the Mellon reproductive biology centers. *Int J Gynaecol Obstet* 67(suppl 2):S101–S110.

McCauley TC, Kurth BE, Norton EJ, Klotz KL, Westbrook VA, Rao AJ, Herr JC, Diekman AB. 2002. Analysis of a human sperm CD52 glycoform in primates: identification of an animal model for immunocontraceptive vaccine development. *Biol Reprod* 66(6):1681–1688.

National Co-ordinating Group for Male Contraceptives. 1978. Gossypol: a new antifertility agent for males. *Chinese Med J* 4:417–428.

Nieschlag E, Anderson RA, Apter D. 2002. Sixth Summit Meeting Consensus: recommendations for regulatory approval for hormonal male contraception. *Int J Androl* 25(6):375.

Recombinant DNA Advisory Committee. 2000. *About the Recombinant DNA Advisory Committee.* [Online]. Available: http://www4.od.nih.gov/oba/rac/aboutrdagt.htm [accessed August 2003].

Schwartz K, Vilquin JT. 2003. Building the translational highway: toward new partnerships between academia and the private sector. *Nat Med* 9(5):493–495.

Shepard DS, Bail RN, Merritt CG. 2003. Cost-effectiveness of USAID's regional program for family planning in West Africa. *Stud Fam Plann* 34(2):117–126.

Sivin I, Greenslade F, Schmidt F, Waldman SN. 1994. *The Copper T380 Intrauterine Device: A Summary of Scientific Data.* New York: The Population Council.

Society for the Advancement of Women's Health Corporate Advisory Council. 1995. *Toward a Women's Health Research Agenda: "Risk and Liability: What Are the Implications for Women's Health Research?"* Washington, DC: Society For the Advancement of Women's Health.

Sukcharoen N, Aribarg A, Kriangsinyos R, Chanprasit Y, Ngeamvijawat J. 1996. Contraceptive efficacy and adverse effects of testosterone enanthate in Thai men. *J Med Assoc Thai* 79(12):767–773.

U.S. Congress. 2001. *Best Pharmaceuticals for Children Act.* [Online]. Available: http://www.fda.gov/opacom/laws/pharmkids/pharmkids.html [accessed August 2003].

United Nations Population Fund. 2003. *Microbicides for HIV protection.* [Online]. Available: http://www.unfpa.org/hiv/strategic/advances2.htm [accessed August 2003].

Waites GM. 2003. Development of methods of male contraception: impact of the World Health Organization Task Force. *Fertil Steril* 80(1):1–15.

World Health Organization (WHO). 2003. *Report of the Standing Committee: Policy and Coordination Meeting (PCC).* [Online]. Available: http://www.who.int/reproductive-health/pcc2003/4_sc_report.pdf [accessed August 2003].

World Health Organization, Department of Reproductive Health and Research. 2000. *Annual Technical Report.* [Online]. Available: http://www.who.int/reproductive-health/pcc2001/Documents/mip%20exsum.pdf [accessed August 2003].

World Health Organization Task Force on Methods for the Regulation of Male Fertility. 1990. Contraceptive efficacy of testosterone-induced azoospermia in normal men. *Lancet* 336(8721):955–959.

APPENDIX A

Examples of Progress and Impediments in Contraceptive Research and Development

This appendix provides an update on some of the targets identified as promising in the 1996 IOM report (Institute of Medicine, 1996) and describes what progress has been made and what impediments still exist. It is not meant to be comprehensive but rather is meant to highlight examples of some of the changes that have taken place since 1996. Specifically, updates on microbicide development, male contraceptives, antiprogestins, and immunocontraception are provided. Table A.1 lists a variety of reversible female contraceptives that have been approved since 1996 or that are currently under development. All of the contraceptives listed are essentially variations of previous methods that have been available for as long 20 to 40 years. Thus far, no truly novel targets that could provide completely new approaches to contraception have advanced to the clinical testing stage.

ADVANCES IN MICROBICIDES AND SPERMICIDES

The worldwide HIV/AIDS epidemic has spurred a great deal of activity in the area of vaginal microbicide development. Microbicides entail a wide variety of formulations that include chemicals, antibodies, or buffers that can prevent the transmission of sexually transmitted infections (STIs) and in many cases that also act as spermicidal contraceptives. Several microbicides are already in clinical trials to test their efficacy in preventing pregnancy and STI transmission, but many others are also at earlier stages of development. Examples of microbicides in development are listed in Table A.2.

163

TABLE A.1 Female Contraceptives: Changes Since 1996

Contraceptive	Type and Use	Effectiveness Rate	Mechanism of Action and Description
Reversible, FDA approved			
Mirena	Levonorgestrel-releasing intrauterine system (LNG IUS).	~ 99% in the first year. Similar in form to a T-shaped IUD. Vertical portion of T bears a small cylinder containing LNG.	LNG renders the endometrium unresponsive to estrogen, which is responsible for growth of uterine lining in preparation for pregnancy. LNG also renders the cervical mucus hostile to sperm penetration, hence preventing fertilization.
NuvaRing	Hormone/ monthly vaginal ring.	98%-99% when used as directed.	The first monthly hormone-releasing vaginal ring used for birth control. A soft, flexible transparent ring ~$1/_8$ inch thick with an outer diameter of 2 inches containing etonorgestrel and ethinyl estradiol. Impedes ovulation and implantation. Unlike Cervical caps and diaphragms, the exact placement in the vagina is not critical for it to be effective. The ring is left in the vagina for 3 weeks, after which it is removed for 1 week and then a new ring is inserted.
Progesterone vaginal ring	Hormone/ vaginal ring.	Over 98.5% when used as directed.	Inhibits cervical mucus production and prevents ovulation in lactating women.
Lunelle	Hormone/ monthly injection.	99%	Combines medoxyprogesterone acetate and estradiol cypionate, which suppress ovulation, thicken the cervical mucus, and thin the endometrium. Intramuscular injections are given by a health care provider every 28 to 30 days.

Development and FDA Approval	Side Effects
Approved by FDA in December 2000 for up to 5 years of use. Approved for 5 years of use in most countries where it is available. Developed by Population Council and manufactured by Schering Oy Laboratories. Distributed in the United States by Berlex Laboratories. Widely used in Europe and developing countries.	Irregular bleeding and amenorrhea, rare hormone-related side effects. Health benefits include reduced number of days of bleeding and increase in hemoglobin levels.
Developed by Organon, Inc. Approved by FDA on October 3, 2001.	Irregular bleeding, weight gain, breast tenderness, nausea, changes in mood.
Approved only in Chile.	Minimal.
Approved by FDA in October 2001. Manufactured by Pharmacia Corporation; the company initiated a voluntary recall October 2002 of Lunelle prefilled syringes because of a lack of assurance of full potency and possible risk of contraceptive failure.	Same as those for combination oral hormonal contraceptives.

continued

TABLE A.1 Continued

Contraceptive	Type and Use	Effectiveness Rate	Mechanism of Action and Description
Implanon	Hormone/ implant.	99%	Implanon is a progestogen-only contraceptive implant; a small, flexible rod, 40 millimeters (mm) long and 2 mm in diameter inserted under the skin on the inside of the upper arm. Contains 68 mg of etonorgestrel released over the 3-year life of the device. Inhibits ovulation and thickens the cervical mucus.
Norplant	Hormone/ implant.	97-99%	Six thin, flexible silicone capsules, 33 mm long and 2.4 mm in diameter, containing 36 mg of LNG, for a total of 216 mg. The capsules are inserted under the skin in a minor surgical procedure; this method is effective for up to 5 years.
Jadelle	Hormone/ implant.	99%	Two flexible silicone rods filled with LNG inserted under the skin (very similar to Norplant). Each Jadelle rod is 43 mm long and 2.5 mm in diameter and contains 5 mg of LNG (total of 150 mg); effective for up to 5 years.
Ortho Evra	Transdermal hormonal system.	99.6% when used as directed.	A transdermal patch is applied each week for 3 weeks and is then removed for 1 week. It uses ethinyl estradiol and norelgestromin.
Depo-Provera	Hormone injection.	97-99% when used as directed.	An intramuscular injection of depo-medroxyprogesterone acetate given every 12 weeks.
Seasonale	Hormonal oral contraceptive	Over 99% when used as directed.	Used for 84 days before a 7-day placebo instead of the usual 21-day/7-day cycle. It contains LNG and ethinyl estradiol.

Development and FDA Approval	Side Effects
FDA approved and marketed by Organon International since 1998.	Irregular bleeding, weight gain, acne, headache, and breast tenderness.
Received FDA approval in 1990 but is no longer available in the United States because Wyeth Ayerst took it off the U.S. market. Norplant has been approved in 58 countries. Developed by Population Council.	Irregular bleeding, headache, weight gain, nausea, and acne.
Received FDA approval in 1996; presently approved for use for up to 5 years. However, it is not yet available in the United States. Developed by the Population Council and manufactured by Schering Oy	Irregular bleeding, weight gain, headaches, acne, and mood changes.
Received FDA approval on November 20, 2001. Produced by Ortho-McNeil.	Same as those for combination oral hormonal contraceptives.
Received FDA approval in 1992, produced by Pfizer.	Amenorrhea.
Developed by Barr Laboratories, Inc. Received FDA approved in September 2003.	Same as those for combination oral hormonal contraceptives.

continued

TABLE A.1 Continued

Contraceptive	Type and Use	Effectiveness Rate	Mechanism of Action and Description
Cyclessa	Hormonal oral contraceptive	Over 99% when used as directed. ~ 93% over 1 year of typical use.	Desogestrel/ethinyl estradiol.
Yasmin	Hormonal oral contraceptive	Over 99% when used as directed. ~93% over 1 year of typical use.	Yasmin is a monophasic birth control pill. Each of the first 21 pills contains the same amount of estrogen (ethinyl estradiol) and progestin (drospirenone).
LNG (Levonorgestrel) Known as Plan B when used for emergency contraception (EC).	Hormonal oral contraceptive	Reduces the risk of pregnancy from ~ 8% to 1.1% following a single act of unprotected sex.	Believed to act as an EC principally by preventing ovulation or fertilization; it may also inhibit implantation, but is not effective once implantation has begun. It is administered within 72 hours of unprotected intercourse for EC as two consecutive doses (12 hours apart) of 0.75 mg of LNG, a totally synthetic progestogen (total dose of 1.5 mg).
LNG and ethinyl estradiol tablets	Emergency oral contraceptive	Combined EC is 75% effective.	LNG and ethinyl estradiol.
Preven Emergency Contraceptive Kit	Emergency oral contraceptive	74% effective (with no contraception, 7.2% pregnancies expected; with Yuzpe method, 1.9% pregnancies expected.)	LNG and ethinyl estradiol. The PREVEN Emergency Contraceptive regimen uses the Yuzpe method. Therapy must be initiated as soon as possible within 72 hours after unprotected intercourse.

Development and FDA Approval	Side Effects
Received FDA approval on December 20, 2000. Developed by Organon, Inc.	Same as those for combination oral hormonal contraceptives.
Received FDA approval in May 2003. Developed by Berlex Laboratories. Yasmin 28 was approved by the FDA on May 2001, and earlier in Europe. Developed by Schering AG.	Same as those for combination oral hormonal contraceptives, except for less bloating than that with other hormonal methods.
FDA approved Plan B in July 1999 for EC following unprotected sex and is currently the only progestin-only EC approved by FDA. Developed by Women's Capital Corporation (WCC) financed largely by foundations and other not-for-profit organizations. WCC submitted an application for nonprescription use to FDA on April 21, 2003; supporting research was conducted by not-for-profit research organizations, including Family Health International (FHI), the University of California at San Francisco, the Children's Hospitals of Los Angeles and Pittsburgh, and the World Health Organization (WHO). Barr Laboratories, Inc., signed a letter of intent in October 2003 to acquire Plan B from the WCC.	Produces much less vomiting and nausea than other ECs containing both progestin and estrogen.
Received FDA approval on April 29, 2003. Developed by Barr Laboratories, Inc.	Vomiting and nausea are potential side effects of EC pills.
FDA approved as of June, 1999. Developed by Gynetics, Inc.	Vomiting and nausea are potential side effects of EC pills.

continued

TABLE A.1 Continued

Contraceptive	Type and Use	Effectiveness Rate	Mechanism of Action and Description
Leah's Shield	Vaginal barrier used with a spermicidal lubricant.	~ 85% over 1 year of use.	One size, reusable vaginal barrier method made of silicone with a cup-shaped design and a valve, and loop for easy removal.
FemCap	Vaginal barrier.	77.2% over 1 year of use.	Silicone rubber cervical cap in three sizes with a brim designed to fit into the vaginal fornices.
SILCS diaphragm	Vaginal barrier.	Not tested yet.	A reusable vaginal barrier in three sizes with a dome that covers the cervix, a rim that fits the vaginal fornices, and a brim that conforms to the vagina.
Reality female condom	Vaginal barrier.	~ 95% when used as directed.	Barrier. Made of plastic polyurethane (stronger than latex).
Today Sponge	Vaginal barrier	89% to 91% when used according to instructions; otherwise use effectiveness rate is 84% to 87%.	The active ingredient in the Today Sponge is nonoxynol-9.

Development and FDA Approval	Side Effects
Developed at Yama Inc. Approved by FDA March 14, 2002. Studies have been conducted collaboratively between CONRAD, Yama, and FHI.	Minimal.
FemCap, Inc., received FDA approval on March 28, 2003. Approved in Europe (EC Certificate No. 99-010901). Available in Germany and Italy.	Minimal.
Developed at Program for Appropriate Technology in Health (PATH) in conjunction with SILCS, Inc. The SILCS device is currently being studied for function, acceptability, and safety.	Minimal.
Collaboration between CONRAD and Medtech Products Ltd. (in India).	Minimal.
FDA application was withdrawn by Whitehall-Robins Healthcare and then filed by another company; Allendale Pharmaceuticals; currently under review by FDA.	Minimal.

continued

TABLE A.1 Continued

Contraceptive	Type and Use	Effectiveness Rate	Mechanism of Action and Description
Examples of Reversible Contraceptives in Development			
Progesterone receptor modulators	Hormonal oral contraceptive but estrogen-free	Unknown	Antigonadotropic. Prevents follicular growth and suppresses ovulation.
Biodegradable implants, for example, Capronor	Hormone-releasing implants	NA	Implants containing progestin are implanted under the skin of the arm or hip. The hormone is released gradually into the body for 12 to 18 months. Capronor II consists of two rods of poly(e-caprolactone), each containing 18 mg of levonorgestrel (LNG). Capronor III is a single capsule of copolymer (caprolactone and trimethylenecarbonate) filled with 32 mg of LNG. With both systems, the implant remains intact during the first year of use and thus could be removed if needed. Over the second year, it biodegrades to carbon dioxide and water, which are absorbed by the body.
GnRH analogs	Could be administered subdermally or other ways.	NA	A new group of drugs known as GnRH antagonists can be used to prevent the release of FSH and LH from the pituitary gland. The release of FSH and LH triggers ovulation and spermatogenesis (the development of sperm). Blocking the release of these hormones temporarily suppresses fertility for women and men.
Nestorone/EE vaginal ring	Female hormonal contraceptive, progestin and estrogen.	Phase II trials indicate over 90% ovulation suppression.	Suppresses follicular growth and ovulation.

Development and FDA Approval	Side Effects

In FDA pipeline.

None has been FDA approved.

One form, Cetrorelix, is approved as a GnRH antagonist for other indications. | First-generation antagonists caused histamine release and local allergic reaction. New analogs are better tolerated.

Developed by the Population Council. Phase II trials completed, phase III trials formulation and manufacture by Q Pharma in Sweden.

continued

TABLE A.1 Continued

Contraceptive	Type and Use	Effectiveness Rate	Mechanism of Action and Description
Frameless IUDs, including Gynefix	IUD	Same rate as other IUDs (~99%).	Similar to regular IUDs but without the rigid frame. It is hoped that they will cause less cramping because there is no rigid frame to press against the uterus. It consists of six copper tubing segments attached to a nylon thread, with a knot at the top end that serves as an anchor. The knot is implanted in the myometrium of the uterine fundus, permanently securing the device in the uterine cavity.
Silicone plugs	Reversible nonsurgical method of tubal sterilization, such as Ovabloc	No pregnancies reported, but 8% experienced migration of the plugs.	A reversible, nonsurgical method of tubal sterilization. Liquid silicone is injected into the fallopian tubes. The silicone hardens and blocks the tube with a rubbery plug that can be removed. Could also be used in males.
Irreversible			
Essure	Nonsurgical sterilization via bilateral occlusion of the fallopian tubes	>99% with successful placement; first procedure placement rate of 86%.	An expandable microcoil insert placed in the fallopian tubes, where it promotes the formation of tissue that blocks the passageway and anchors the device permanently in place. Insertion procedure does not require an incision in the abdominal cavity and can be performed under local anesthesia.
Chemical scarring	Nonsurgical sterilization	NA	Two different chemical combinations can be used to achieve scarring that eventually blocks the fallopian tubes: phenol (carbolic acid) with a thickening agent or phenol with quinacrine

Development and FDA Approval	Side Effects
In European clinical trials. Available in the United Kingdom since 1998.	The frameless IUDs occasionally have problems with early expulsion, though Gynefix is said to have a lower rate of expulsion.
Studies are under way in the Netherlands. Used by men in China. Not FDA approved.	Unknown.
Received FDA approval in September 2002. Manufactured by Conceptus.	Discomfort on day of insertion.
Quinacrine is used in China; not approved by any regulatory body; recommended to be further tested in studies with animals before any further use in humans.	Cancer risk, potential damage to a fetus if inadvertently administered to a pregnant woman, and increased risk of ectopic pregnancy.

continued

TABLE A.1 Continued

Contraceptive	Type and Use	Effectiveness Rate	Mechanism of Action and Description
Chemical plugs	Nonsurgical sterilization.	NA	Introduction of chemicals, such as methylcyanoacrylate (MCA), into the fallopian tubes.
Cryosurgery	Nonsurgical sterilization.	NA	Liquid nitrogen is used to freeze the cornua; scar tissue blocks the fallopian tubes.

NOTE: NA = not available.
GENERAL SOURCES:
 FHI (http://www.fhi.org/en/RH/Pubs/Network/v18_1/NW181ch5.htm)
 FDA (http://www.fda.gov/)
 U.S. Patent and Trademark Office (http://www.uspto.gov/)
 Planned Parenthood Federation of America (http://www.plannedparenthood.org/),
  especially (http://www.plannedparenthood.org/ARTICLES/bcfuture_w.html)
 Geneva Foundation for Medical Education and Research (http://www.gfmer.ch/)
 Reproductive Health Online, from Johns Hopkins University
  (http://www.reproline.jhu.edu/)
 Population Council, New York, NY (http://www.popcouncil.org/)

Development and FDA Approval	Side Effects
Approved in Canada and the Netherlands.	

Trussell and Vaughn, 1999
Product sites:
Yasmin (http://www.yasmin.com)
Today Sponge (http://www.todaysponge.com/)
Company sites:
Barr Laboratories (http://www.barrlabs.com/home.html)
Progesterone ring:
Massai et al., 2000; Sivin et al. 1997

TABLE A.2 Examples of Microbicides and Spermicides in Development

Microbicide	Type and Use	Effectiveness Rate	Mechanism of Action and Description
Examples of microbicides with spermicidal activity			
BufferGel (Carbopol polymer)	Microbicide; buffered gel. Nonirritating lubricant made of a Carbopol gel (Carbopol 974P), which is a high-molecular-weight, cross-linked polyacrylic acid. It contains no oil or detergent and is compatible for use with condoms and latex diaphragms.	Unknown; potential spermicide and protection against STIs.	Maintains the natural acidity of the vagina, even in the presence of seminal fluid, and creates a physical barrier that inhibits the passage of pathogens into the vaginal and cervical epithelium.
Savvy (C31G)	Microbicide; surfactant. Designed to be applied vaginally before sexual intercourse. It is also a spermicide.	Unknown.	Equimolar mixture of the amphoteric surfactants cetyl betaine and myristamine oxide; surfactant/detergent that kills or disables pathogens by stripping them of their outer covering.
Ushercell (cellulose sulfate)	Microbicide gel; adsorption inhibitor.	Unknown; in vitro and animal studies have shown that Ushercell is a potent contraceptive and microbicide.	High-molecular-weight cellulose sulfate compound. Prevents pathogens from adhering to and eventually passing through the walls of healthy cells.

Stage of Development and FDA Approval	Side Effects
Developed by ReProtect LLC and Johns Hopkins University with support from NICHD and the HIV Prevention Trials Network (HPTN). Two clinical trials for safety and side effects with 27 women in the United States and 98 women in four other countries have been conducted. Two smaller clinical trials have shown BufferGel to be safe and nonirritating to men. Data from phase II/III trial on BufferGel's contraceptive activity are expected in 2004; data on the anti-HIV activity of BufferGel are expected in 2006.	In a phase I trial, mild vaginal itching and irritation. Vaginal candidiasis and hyperkeratotic lesions required discontinuation of the product in a small percentage of trial participants. An international phase I clinical trial had similar results. Adverse events were categorized as mild to moderate, and included *Candida* on wet mount, vaginal/vulval itching or burning after insertion or when passing urine, labial rash, lower abdominal pain, and vaginal discharge.
In 2002, with support from NICHD, Biosyn successfully completed two phase I/II safety and efficacy studies for C31G vaginal gel, a dose escalation study, and a postcoital testing (PCT) study for contraceptive efficacy. C31G is now positioned to enter phase III clinical trials for contraception and the prevention of HIV, herpes simplex virus, and chlamydia infections and gonorrhea.	
Developed by Polydex Pharmaceuticals (Canada) and the Program for the Topical Prevention of Conception and Disease (TOPCAD; Chicago, IL). As of September 2002, Ushercell has completed three phase I/II clinical trials of safety, acceptability, and male tolerance of 6% gel. Other phase I/II clinical trials are planned and ongoing. Phase III human clinical trials are planned for fiscal year 2004 under the direction of CONRAD.	

continued

TABLE A.2 Continued

Microbicide	Type and Use	Effectiveness Rate	Mechanism of Action and Description
ACIDFORM	Microbicide; buffered gel. Designed to be applied vaginally before sexual intercourse.	Unknown; potential spermicide and protection against STIs.	Has no active ingredient but is a combination of compounds that work together to maintain the natural protective acidity of the normal vaginal environment, even in the presence of alkaline semen. Maintains low vaginal pH, which immobilizes sperm and should prevent multiplication and survival of sexually transmitted pathogens.
Praneem	Spermicide. Contains purified extracts from the neem tree combined with citrata oil.	Unknown.	Mechanism is unknown or uncharacterized.

Examples of microbicides with no known spermicidal activity

Microbicide	Type and Use	Effectiveness Rate	Mechanism of Action and Description
Carraguard (formerly known as PC-515)	Microbicide in aqueous solution; adsorption inhibitor. Designed to be applied vaginally before sexual intercourse.	Assumed to be non-contraceptive on the basis of laboratory work.	Fusion inhibitor; it provides a physical barrier that keeps HIV and other pathogens from reaching target cells.
Emmelle (dextrin sulfate)	Microbicide gel; adsorption inhibitor. Icodextrin-based intravaginal gel to prevent HIV infection.	Not known to be effective as a contraceptive.	A phase I trial of safety with males has been completed. Phase I and II trials of safety and dosage have been completed. Phase III clinical trial to be conducted in Africa is being planned (M-L Laboratories).
Lactin vaginal capsule	Microbicide.	Unknown.	Recolonizes the vagina with *Lactobacillus* to maintain vaginal acidity.

Stage of Development and FDA Approval	Side Effects
Instead Inc. licensed from Rush Medical Center (TOPCAD) in February 2003. Two phase I safety studies were completed by the Global Microbicide Project (GMP); an acceptability trial for use with diaphragm is planned for 2004.	
Phase I trials at the Institute of Research and Reproduction, India	Unknown.
Developed by the Population Council, with funding from CDC, USAID, and the Gates Foundation. Several phase I and II trials of Carraguard and earlier forms of carrageenan-based microbicides were completed; phase III effectiveness trials will begin in January 2004.	No side effects mentioned. Phase II trials have shown Carraguard to be safe when taken vaginally for up to 12 months.
Developer: M-L Laboratories in the United Kingdom. Phase II trials supported by the Medical Research Council, United Kingdom, Institute of Tropical Medicine, Belgium	
Phase II trials at the University of Pittsburgh sponsored by NIAID	

continued

TABLE A.2 Continued

Microbicide	Type and Use	Effectiveness Rate	Mechanism of Action and Description
Polystyrene sulfonate	Microbicide gel; adsorption inhibitor. Designed to be applied vaginally before sexual intercourse.	Unknown.	
PRO 2000 (naphthalene 2-sulfonate polymer)	Microbicide gel; adsorption inhibitor. Designed to be applied vaginally before sexual intercourse.	Unknown; potential efficacy demonstrated in rabbits.	Unlike other sulfonated polymers, such as dextran sulfate, which act by binding to the V3 loop of glycoprotein gp120, PRO 2000 also binds to CD4 cells and interferes with the gp120–CD4 interaction. It provides a physical barrier that keeps HIV and other pathogens from reaching the target cells.
SAMMA (mandelic acid condensation polymer)	Microbicide gel; adsorption inhibitor. Designed to be applied vaginally before sexual intercourse.	Unknown.	In vitro tests found that mandelic acid condensation polymer inhibits sperm function (but does not kill sperm).
Tenofovir PMPA gel	Microbicide gel.	Non-spermicidal.	Non-nucleoside reverse transcriptase inhibitor; interferes with transcription of viral RNA to DNA.

SOURCES:

http://www.itg.be/micro2002/downloads/presentations/2Monday_May_13_2002/
    Track_B_C_session/Polly_Harrison.pdf
http://www.aegis.com/news/bw/2003/BW030206.html
http://www.aidsmap.com/web/pb1/eng/EF5AB676-885A-4F55-8912-9DD1FE9BEE92.htm
http://www.mihivnews.com/microbicides-news.htm
http://www.agi-usa.org/pubs/journals/gr040501.html

Stage of Development and FDA Approval	Side Effects

A phase I safety study has been completed; expanded safety studies are planned. Sponsored by GMP.

Clinical trials undertaken by NIH, HPTN, and Indevus Pharmaceuticals. Phase I clinical trials, conducted in Europe, found that PRO 2000 was well tolerated by healthy, sexually abstinent women. Findings from a phase I/II trial, conducted in the United States and South Africa, indicate a similarly promising safety profile in healthy, sexually active women. PRO 2000 has been selected for testing in a large phase II/III pivotal trial to assess safety and protective efficacy. This trial will involve women in the United States, India, and several African countries.

A few non-HIV-positive male patients reported mild symptoms of genital itching, tingling, irritation, dryness, discoloration, or flaking of the dried gel.

Preclinical studies at Rush-Presbyterian-St. Luke's Medical Center, Chicago.

Unknown.

Unknown.

http://www.niaid.nih.gov/daids/prevention/text/microbes.htm
http://www.global-campaign.org/clientfiles/PipelineFactsheet.pdf
http://www.global-campaign.org/clientfiles/cone.pdf
http://www.rhtp.org/micro/micro_research_pipeline.htm
http://www.popcouncil.org/biomed/microbicides.html
Amaral et al., 1999; Garg et al., 2001

The development of an effective contraceptive microbicide presents an enormous challenge in that it must be highly effective against pathogens and sperm, but it must not disrupt the normal flora or mucosal cells of the vagina even when it is used very frequently. In addition, establishing evidence of efficacy requires multiple clinical trials with different populations to test both the efficacy of the microbicide as a contraceptive and the efficacy of the microbicide for protection against specific STIs. Thus, the clinical testing stage is a very expensive, time-consuming process. To complicate matters, the Food and Drug Administration (FDA) has not provided guidance on how best to test the safety and efficacy of microbicides in clinical trials. At a recent meeting of an FDA advisory panel, the group discussed whether tests of microbicides should compare the product to condom use or to an inactive placebo, or both. The group also discussed how long an experimental microbicide trial should be and what data would need to be reported to show that the microbicide was effective. However, the panel was unable to come to a consensus on the issues and noted that the first experimental microbicide to be tested would likely face many obstacles (Kaisernetwork, 2003).

Recently, the field has been energized by an influx of new funding from nonfederal and federal sources and by the establishment of several new initiatives or organizations. For example, the Global Microbicide Project (Global Microbicide Project, 2000)[1] was established in 2000 to help develop new microbicidal agents that specifically address the needs and perspectives of women. The main objective of this project is to develop vaginal methods that would protect women against STIs including HIV/ AIDS. Funding for GMP comes solely from the Bill and Melinda Gates Foundation to expedite microbicide development. Additional funding to investigate the contraceptive efficacy of microbicides is available through the Consortium for Industrial Collaboration in Contraceptive Research (CICCR). GMP can provide funds for both pilot and major projects. Although there is no requirement for cost sharing by an industrial partner, it is strongly encouraged. There is no limit to funding for a project, but initial funding for a new project may be limited in time and amount until the feasibility of the proposed approach has been determined. Recently, the U.S. Agency for International Development has also provided significant sums of money to the Population Council, Family Health International, and CONRAD (the parent organization of GMP and CICCR) for microbicide development.

Support from other foundations may also speed progress in the field. The International Partnership for Microbicides (International Partnership

---

[1]See http://www.gmp.org/ (accessed September 2003).

for Microbicides, 2002) was established in 2002 as a result of a study supported by the Rockefeller Foundation. IPM acts as a coordinating body and central repository of funds, with the goal of accelerating progress in the microbicide field.

The formation of the Alliance for Microbicide Development has been credited with driving progress in the field as well. Founded in 1998, the Alliance[2] is a global, not-for-profit organization whose sole mission is to speed the development of safe, effective, and affordable microbicides to prevent STIs, most critically, HIV/AIDS. The Alliance defines itself as a catalyst, communicator, convener, and problem solver. It consists of a global coalition of representatives from more than 200 biopharmaceutical companies, not-for-profit research institutions, and health advocacy groups. As such, it provides authoritative information on microbicide development, facilitates dialogue on key policy issues, provides education about the public health potential of microbicides, and serves as an advocate for the resources needed to develop them. The work of the Alliance is funded by contributions from the William and Flora Hewlett Foundation, the International Partnership for Microbicides, the Moriah Fund, the Rockefeller Foundation, the Bill and Melinda Gates Foundation through GMP, and a number of private contributors. Other areas of contraceptive research would likely also benefit from the establishment of similar entities that could serve as information sources and activity coordinators.

UPDATE ON MALE CONTRACEPTION

Hormonal Methods

Before the 1960s, when oral contraceptives and intrauterine devices (IUDs) were introduced, the most commonly used contraception methods—condoms and withdrawal—were male directed. Even now, contraceptive use among men, which is essentially limited to condoms and vasectomy, accounts for nearly one-third of all current contraceptive use in the United States and worldwide (Meriggiola et al., 2003). Surveys performed in recent years also suggest that the majority of men are willing to share the responsibility for family planning and that women in stable relationships would trust their male partner to use contraceptives (Glasier et al., 2000; Martin et al., 2000; Weston et al., 2002).

The potential for hormonal contraception for men has been recognized for more than 50 years, and a number of regimens have been tested in the clinic, but to date, none has been submitted for FDA review or approved

---

[2]http://www.microbicide.org/ (accessed August 2003).

for use in other countries. (See Table A.3 for examples of male contraceptives in development.) Significant efforts have been devoted to the development of male hormonal contraceptives over the last several decades. However, progress has been quite slow for a variety of reasons, including sporadic funding, limited interest by pharmaceutical companies, and at times, political and cultural concerns (Meriggiola et al., 2003; reviewed by Waites, 2003). An additional impediment may be the lack of regulatory guidelines on the requirement for demonstrating the safety and efficacy of male contraceptives (Nieschlag et al., 2002). Nonetheless, the World Health Organization (WHO) and CONRAD have been major forces in moving the field forward. A number of male-directed methods are in clinical trials, and at least one (testosterone undecanoate [TU]) appears to be close to achieving registration for use in China (Waites, 2003). Several others (Table A.3) are at earlier stages of development but show significant promise (Meriggiola et al., 2003; Waites, 2003).

Reversibility is the primary attraction of hormonal methods. Approximately 3,000 men have participated in clinical trials of male hormonal contraceptive methods over the last 20 years, and none of them has failed to return their sperm counts to normal and eventual fertility.[3] One limitation of such methods is the slow onset and offset of action—from 1 to 4 months—because of the hormones' delayed effects on spermatogenesis in the testes. A further incentive for development is the theoretical possibility that some of these agents could eventually decrease the risk of some diseases, such as prostate disease. They might also possibly result in a decreasing rate of baldness, which, although not a health issue, might be important in terms of acceptance. Long-term effects on health, however, are unknown.

The three formulations currently used in the development of male hormonal contraceptives are testosterone alone, testosterone plus progestins, and testosterone plus gonadotropin-releasing hormone (GnRH) antagonists. All of these agents exploit the same basic mechanism. They inhibit the central stimulatory pathways for gonadotropin production, which leads to the suppression of Leydig cell function and testosterone secretion and, thus, to decreased sperm production in the testes. Exogenous testosterone replaces the suppressed endogenous testosterone, which is necessary to maintain libido and well-being.

The administration of testosterone alone can produce azoospermia in some men, but this approach has been plagued by considerable variability in response. For example, in an early WHO study of couples, only 65

---

[3]William J. Bremner, University of Washington, in a presentation at the International Symposium on New Frontiers in Contraceptive Research, Washington, DC, July 15-16, 2003.

percent of the participating men developed azoospermia (World Health Organization Task Force on Methods for the Regulation of Male Fertility, 1990). There was, however, a very low birth rate in the group because the majority of men experienced oligospermia (abnormally low sperm counts). A later WHO trial documented a total failure rate for testosterone of about 3 to 4 percent (World Health Organization Task Force on Methods for the Regulation of Male Fertility, 1996), which is comparable to the failure rates that are often reported for female methods. This failure rate is vastly better than that reported for the condoms, which would be the appropriate direct comparison for these methods.

High-dose testosterone had some side effects, such as increased muscle mass and weight, with a corresponding decrease in fat mass, but these were not viewed as adverse events. Some participants experienced an increase in oily skin and acne, and there was also about a 10 percent decrease in high-density lipoprotein (HDL) levels.[4] About 25 percent of the men experienced a decrease in testicular size as well.

Other traditional androgens are also being tested as single-agent contraceptives. TU has been available as an oral preparation for decades and has been used, primarily by the Chinese, in oil as an injectable preparation. In a recent efficacy study in China, 299 of 308 men achieved either azoospermia or had counts low enough to enter an efficacy phase of the study (Gu et al., 2003). There was only one pregnancy among couples who were using TU as the sole means of contraception for 1 year, and no serious side effects were reported.

Researchers are also exploring whether the addition of progestins to testosterone can lead to a more effective contraceptive. Formulations have included depot medroxyprogesterone acetate (DMPA); levonorgestrel (either orally or in implants); desogesterol and its in vivo metabolite, etonorgestrel (in an implant made by Organon); and cyproterone acetate (CPA; which is taken orally).

In one study, which compared testosterone alone to the same dose of testosterone enanthate combined with oral levonorgestrel, the progestin showed a clear additive effect on the rapidity and completeness of suppression of sperm production compared with the effect of testosterone alone (Bebb et al., 1996). In a study of CPA plus testosterone compared with testosterone alone, the progestin again increased the rapidity and completeness of suppression of sperm production, and at higher doses all men achieved azoospermia (Meriggiola et al., 1996).

Testosterone has also been combined with GnRH antagonists. GnRH

---

[4]It is not known whether this has the same risk that is associated with spontaneous low HDL levels.

TABLE A.3 Examples of Male Contraceptives in Development

Contraceptive	Type and Use	Effectiveness Rate	Mechanism of Action and Description
Cystatin 11	Epididymal protein.		
Depo-medroxy-progesterone acetate (DMPA)	Hormonal suppression of sperm production. Used in combination with some form of testosterone replacement.	No pregnancy in 55 couples treated with DMPA + testosterone pellets every 3 to 4 months.	Long-acting progestin, Antigonadotropic agent, blocks LH and FSH production and hence sperm production.
Eppin	Immuno-contraceptive.	Unknown.	Stimulates immune system to inactivate an epididymal enzyme that plays a role in sperm maturation.
GnRH coupled with protein	Immuno-contraceptive.	Unknown.	Stimulates immune system to inactivate the body's natural GnRH, suppressing sperm production.
Lonidamine (LND) derivatives	Male nonhormonal contraceptive.	Unknown.	Understanding is incomplete; causes premature release of germ cells from the testis by action on the adherens junctions between Sertoli and germ cells.
MENT (7-α-methyl-19-nortestosterone)	Synthetic hormone resembling testosterone; implanted under the skin of a man's upper arm (a transdermal gel is used in aging males).	Nine of 11 men in a dosage trial had zero sperm counts after four implants.	Antigonadotropic and androgen replacement.

Stage of Development and FDA Approval	Side Effects
Studies with primates are planned.	
	Androgen deficiency (requiring that testosterone pellets are also used); delay of up to 7 months before recovery of spermatogenesis.
Promising results from studies with primates.	Unknown.
In early stages of research.	Unknown.
Approved for use as an anticancer drug. Population Council developed two synthetic analogs that are antispermatogenetic and nontoxic in rats. Results of tests of toxicity at low doses over long periods of time are pending.	
In the FDA pipeline. Developed by the Population Council and Schering AG	No effect on the prostate.

continued

TABLE A.3 Continued

Contraceptive	Type and Use	Effectiveness Rate	Mechanism of Action and Description
Testosterone buciclate (TB)	Male hormonal contraceptive; androgen. Injected every 3 months.	68% responded.	Suppresses GnRH secretion and thus sperm production.
Testosterone enanthate (TE)	Male hormonal contraceptive; androgen. Injected; potent for 10 days.		Suppresses GnRH secretion and thus sperm production.
Testosterone undecanoate (TU)	Male hormonal contraceptive; androgen.		Suppresses GnRH secretion and thus sperm production.
Vasclip	Vasectomy alternative; should be considered permanent.	97.5%	Polymeric clip occludes vas deferens to prevent sperm flow.
Reversible inhibition of sperm under guidance (RISUG)	Vas deferens occlusion by styrene maleic anhydride (SMA) complexed with the solvent dimethyl sulfoxide.	Reported to be 100% when correctly inserted in vas deferens, in small studies.	SMA complex is injected into the vasa deferentia by a no-scalpel procedure. The positive and negative charge mosaic causes the membranes of passing sperm to rupture.

SOURCES:

Cheng et al. (2001), Gatto et al. (2002), Gupta (2003), Mishra et al. (2003), World Health
  Organization Task Force on Methods for the Regulation of Male Fertility (1990)
  http://www.popcouncil.org/biomed/malecontras.html
  http://www.reproline.jhu.edu/
  http://www.engenderhealth.org/wh/fp/ceff.html#barrier

Stage of Development and FDA Approval	Side Effects
	Oily skin, aggressiveness, increased muscle mass, decreased HDL levels.
One of the earliest treatments for hypogonadism, researched as a male hormonal contraceptive since the 1970s.	Similar to those of other androgens.
Efficacy study in China.	Similar to those of other androgens.
Approved by FDA in August 2002. Now available in the United States. Expected launch in Europe by January 2004.	Pain during procedure, although significantly reduced pain and complications compared with those after a traditional vasectomy.
Phase I and phase II trials completed in India. Currently in phase III clinical trials.	Because RISUG does not completely block the flow of sperm through the vas deferens, it appears not to have any of the negative side effects associated with vasectomies. Lack of toxicity remains to be confirmed.

http://www.reproline.jhu.edu/english/6read/6issues/6network/v18-3/nt1835a.html
http://www.avert.org/condoms.htm#2
http://www.popcouncil.org/publications/popbriefs/pb8(2)_4.html
http://www.malecontraceptives.org/methods/risug.htm

antagonists block the effect of GnRH coming from the hypothalamus to the pituitary gland and thereby decrease the production of luteinizing hormone (LH) and follicle-stimulating hormone (FSH), which reduces the levels of testosterone and sperm production. This approach has been shown in small pilot studies in the United States and Europe to be an effective method, although it has not been determined how long this suppression can be maintained, and larger follow-up studies are needed (Swerdloff et al., 1998). To avoid undesirable side effects, GnRH antagonists cannot be used in isolation. Testosterone is a necessary adjunct for the long-term use of such antagonists. This combination can be used to achieve azoospermia in a variety of ways, but one approach is to use a GnRH antagonist like acyline for a brief period—such as 12 weeks—at the initiation of a regimen to help with suppression of sperm production and then to stop the antagonist and use testosterone enanthate alone.

Nonhormonal Methods

Various orally active nonhormonal agents have been found in animal models to interfere with spermatogenesis without reducing testosterone levels. Lonidamine is a nonsteroidal, nonhormonal antispermatogenic agent that acts by premature exfoliation of germ cells from the seminiferous epithelium (De Martino et al., 1981; Silvestrini et al., 1984). Although this was a novel mode of action, lonidamine was not developed as a male contraceptive because of its toxic effects on the liver and kidney, but it was used as an antitumor agent (Silvestrini, 1991; Silvestrini et al., 1984). More recently, analogs of lonidamine were discovered that appeared to have the same action on the testes, but apparently without the toxicity of lonidamine (Cheng et al., 2001, 2002; Grima et al., 2001). The Population Council, with the assistance of CICCR, the Mellon Foundation, and the National Institute of Child Health and Human Development (NICHD), has been working on the lead analog AF2364.

Certain hexahyrdoindenopyridines have been reported to act as reversible male contraceptive agents (Cook et al., 1997). A 28-day toxicity study with rats did not reveal any significant toxicity but did confirm the male contraceptive effect (Fail et al., 2000). CICCR is discussing with the Research Triangle Institute the possibility of supporting some further studies with one of the lead compounds in this series, and it is hoped that collaboration with a pharmaceutical company will be possible.

Lastly, a recent report has described the contraceptive activity of alkylated imino sugars in male mice (van der Spoel et al., 2002). When the lead compound, N-butyldeoxynojirimycin, was given orally, epididymal sperm had abnormal head shapes and lacked acrosomal antigens. The motility of the affected spermatozoa was abnormal, and the mice became infertile after 3 weeks of dosing. Fertility was regained in the fourth week after dosing ceased. This compound appeared to exert its effect through interference with the biosynthesis of glucosylceramide-based sphingolipids. These investigators are planning to develop this lead compound further. These are examples of exciting new contraceptive agents already at the proof-of-concept stage and merit further support as potential second-generation nonhormonal male contraceptives.

UPDATE ON ANTIPROGESTINS AS FEMALE HORMONAL CONTRACEPTIVES

The first antiprogestin was discovered in 1980. Since then, more than 400 compounds with antiprogestin activities have been synthesized (Hodgen, 1991), but only a handful have been tested with humans, including mifepristone (formerly Roussel-Uclaf, now Exelgene), onapristone and lilopristone (Schering AG), Org 31710 and Org 31806 (Organon, Inc.), and CDB 2914 (developed by NICHD).

Antiprogestins can affect reproductive function because they bind to progesterone receptors in the hypothalamus, anterior pituitary, and uterus; and in doing so, they inhibit transcription of the genes that are normally activated by progesterone. In other words, the antiprogestins act as receptor antagonists. The contraceptive effects of antiprogestins depend on the dose and the time of the ovarian cycle at which they are administered. Various regimens of mifepristone have been tested, including a single postcoital dose for emergency contraception, as well as daily, weekly, and monthly regimens for conventional contraception (reviewed by Glasier, 2002). The theoretical advantages of weekly or monthly regimes include exposure to lower total doses of the drug, but a disadvantage may be the difficulty in remembering to take the drug at the appropriate time. In each case, inhibition of ovulation or significant disruption of endometrial development, or both, is thought to contribute to contraceptive efficacy.

The contraceptive effects of mifepristone have been demonstrated most clearly in trials of emergency contraception. A single dose of 10, 50, or 600 milligrams (mg) of mifepristone each appears to be equally effective in preventing pregnancy, even up to 120 hours after intercourse (Task Force on Postovulatory Methods of Fertility Regulation, 1999). The mode of action of mifepristone when it is used as an emergency contraceptive depends on the stage of the menstrual cycle when it is taken. Given before ovulation, it prevents ovulation from occurring. Given after ovulation, the effect on the endometrium is indicative of impaired implantation.

For the daily regimen, doses of mifepristone from 10 mg down to 0.1 mg have been tested. Doses between 2 and 10 mg daily have all been shown to inhibit ovulation (Brown et al., 2002; Cameron et al., 1995; Croxatto et al., 1993; Ledger et al., 1992). Sixty-five percent of women taking 2 mg/day and 88 percent of those taking 5 mg/day experienced amenorrhea. Although follicular activity continued during treatment, endometrial development was altered by doses ranging from 0.5 to 10 mg, suggesting that even if ovulation did occur, implantation would have been very unlikely. The contraceptive efficacy of daily low-dose mifepristone has been demonstrated in only two studies. In a study from Scotland and China (with 5 mg of mifepristone), 50 women used no other method of contraception and there were no pregnancies (Brown et al., 2002). In a study of 32 women using 0.5 mg of mifepristone daily, 16 women completed 6 months of use. In 141 cycles, there were five pregnancies (Marions et al., 1999).

In tests of mifepristone administered once per week, doses of 10 to 50 mg were associated with variable inhibition of ovulation (Chen and Xiao, 1997; Spitz et al., 1996), whereas doses of 5 and 2.5 mg did not inhibit ovulation (Gemzell-Danielsson et al., 1996). However, all doses affected endometrial development. The efficacy of a weekly regimen has been tested in only one study involving 18 women (Marions et al., 1998). In that study, three pregnancies occurred over 63 cycles.

The administration of mifepristone once per month is thought to prevent pregnancy by inhibiting implantation. A number of studies have demonstrated that 200 mg of mifepristone given in the early luteal phase slows endometrial development without altering the timing of the next menses. Two studies have demonstrated greater than 95 percent contraceptive efficacy of 200 mg of mifepristone given within 2 days of the LH surge (Gemzell-Danielsson et al., 1993; Hapangama et al., 2001). The limiting factor to this approach is the accurate detection of the LH surge, as the timing of mifepristone administration is critical.

A few other antiprogestins have been tested in studies with humans as well, but much less extensively than mifepristone. Onapristone and lilopristone (Schering AG, Berlin) were both tested for their potential effects on reproductive function in humans, but onapristone was abandoned after phase I studies demonstrated changes in liver function, and lilopristone has not been taken forward. Organon has published data on two antiprogestins, Org 31710 and Org 31806 (Kloosterboer et al., 1994), but clinical testing has not progressed past a very early stage. CDB 2914, which is structurally and functionally similar to mifepristone, has been shown to have no adverse effects in normally cycling women at doses of up to 200 mg (Passaro et al., 1997; Stratton et al., 2000). A clinical trial of this compound as an emergency contraceptive has been completed and results are undergoing analysis.

A new group of compounds called mesoprogestins has also been synthesized and characterized by Jenapharm GmbH & Co. (Jena, Germany). These compounds bind strongly to the progesterone receptor but have mixed agonistic and antagonistic activities in vivo (Chwalisz et al., 2000). Their antiproliferative effects on the endometrium are being investigated in studies with animal models, including primates, but no studies with humans have yet been published.

Although antiprogestins have significant potential for contraceptive development, progress has been hindered by the political controversy surrounding mifepristone, which is licensed in many parts of the world as an abortifacient for use during early pregnancy. Lobbying efforts by groups opposed to abortion have led to limited interest and activity in the development of contraceptive antiprogestins by both the pharmaceutical industry and not-for-profit organizations, despite their potential for preventing unplanned pregnancy.

UPDATE ON IMMUNOCONTRACEPTION

The development of contraceptive vaccines has been pursued since the early days of contraceptive research, but progress in this field has been exceedingly slow, and the work has yet to produce a vaccine that is proven safe and effective for use in humans. Although various investigators had immunized animals with reproductive antigens since the early 1960s, the field of immunocontraception for humans was really launched as a result of a special consultation convened by WHO in Boston in 1973. This was followed by a symposium, Immunological Approaches to Fertility Control, the seventh in the series of Karolinska Symposia on Research Methods in Reproductive Endocrinology (1974). Exploratory studies funded by WHO were undertaken to assess the feasibility of such an approach. WHO then held a symposium in Varna, Bulgaria, in 1975. Papers dealing with different potential antigens, including sperm, eggs, and hormones of the trophoblast, were presented and published (1975). Consideration was also given to the safety of such approaches. Three main considerations that are critical to the success of such an immunological approach are the length of time that antibodies will be effective, the reversibility of the immunocontraceptive, and the hypothetical potential for teratogenicity during periods when antibody levels are declining. At the time, there was great enthusiasm for a vaccine approach, which was novel and different from available contraceptive approaches, and WHO was supporting the work of about 30 scientists.

Use of the β chain of human chorionic gonadotropin (βhCG) was considered to be the most promising lead at the time. Use of the whole βhCG subunit to immunize female baboons showed that antibodies were produced and pregnancy was prevented. A group in India pursued the use of the whole β chain conjugated to tetanus toxoid. After appropriate safety tests, this preparation was administered to women, and it was found that when the circulating antibody was above a threshold value, women were protected from pregnancy; but some women did not respond, and characteristics that would predict a lack of response could not be identified beforehand. This threw into question the practicality of a method in which antibody levels would have to be assessed at regular intervals. Another disadvantage of this approach was that antibodies were also raised against the β subunit of LH (βLH), and from a long-term perspective this was believed to be unsafe. WHO therefore concentrated on only small pieces of the βhCG protein that were not present in βLH, but ensuring a good antibody response to these small peptides has proved difficult.

In the intervening years, the WHO Task Force on Immunological Approaches to Fertility Control continued to support work in this field, but because of unsatisfactory results and declining funding, most leads were abandoned; the βhCG approach was not, however. Delays occurred because of difficulties in selection of adjuvants[5] and delivery vehicles that did not cause local reactions. Nonetheless, an application was submitted to the regulatory authorities in Sweden in May 2002 to carry out a phase I clinical trial with the current formulation of the βhCG immunocontraceptive. A manufacturer of the immunocontraceptive that meets Good Manufacturing Practice standards has been identified, and preparation of clinical supplies of the formulation awaits funding. Lack of funding has also delayed the planned safety studies to be run concurrently with the phase I trial.

The anti-hCG approach still appears to be the most practical because of several very attractive features. First, hCG has a clearly defined biological function that depends on its secretion into the maternal circulation, where it is readily accessible to antibodies. Circulating antibodies can act on the circulating hormone, and one does not have to be concerned with raising adequate antibody levels in an organ such as the fallopian tube or the uterus, which would be the case with many other potential antigens. High levels of pregnancy prevention have been observed in baboons and women if titers are high enough. The trial in India demonstrated that an antibody titer of 50 nanograms per milliliter (ng/ml) was effective in preventing pregnancy. The antibody response declined with time, and fertility was regained when titers fell below 35 ng/ml (Talwar et al., 1994). Second, there is evidence from a study carried out in many developed countries that showed that women wanted a long-acting method that was

---

[5]A substance that is added to a vaccine to improve the immune response so that less vaccine is needed to produce more antibodies.

not permanent but that could be taken without the knowledge of others, especially if it did not cause any endocrine or other metabolic disturbances, had no overt signs of being used, and did not need storage or disposal. An hCG immunocontraceptive meets all of these criteria, which is not true of most other methods. Given the past results, it is likely that booster vaccinations would be needed every 2 to 3 months to maintain adequate antibody responses, but it is known from use of hormonal injectable contraception in women that even monthly injections can be acceptable in some settings (Snow et al., 1997). The production of inexpensive, home-use diagnostic kits would circumvent the problems of assessing antibody levels in cases where the actual titer was critical for contraception by allowing women to determine when the titer is too low to be effective. Such a kit could also screen out the nonresponders. Third, if reversibility became an issue in a small percentage of women, administration of exogenous progesterone to maintain the pregnancy is a potential solution.

However, despite the promise and potential, the project is still at the early clinical trial stage some 30 years after work on this concept began. Some might question whether the work on βhCG should be terminated, since the immunocontraceptive has not reached fruition in 30 years. On the other hand, 20 years of research and substantially greater funding have been devoted to the development of an anti-HIV vaccine, without success to date. The case for continued work on immunocontraceptives has recently been cogently put forth by Aitken (2002). New funding sources, perhaps developed through grass-roots lobbying from consumers wanting different options, could potentially spur progress of the immunocontraceptive approach. The Alliance for Microbicide Development could serve as an instructive model in that regard.

Other targets and formulations for contraceptive vaccines are also under investigation, but thus far, proof of concept has not been firmly established (reviewed by Gupta, 2003). Because immunocontraception could provide an alternative and novel method of fertility regulation, funding should be made available to establish proofs of concept for the most advanced and promising leads, based on sound science, to move the field forward. Examples include sperm surface antigens and epididymal carbohydrate antigens, as well as antigens known to induce immune responses in infertile couples (see the section on proteomics in Chapter 2 for more detail). In the ovum, the oolemma (vitelline membrane) might also be a viable target, although little is known about the oolemma, and such research would be at a much earlier stage than the stages of the approaches noted above.

One challenge for these alternate approaches is accurate assessment of the immune status of those vaccinated. If antibodies are raised to inhibit circulating hormones such as hCG, measurement of the antibody levels is meaningful, but when the level of antibody needs to be high in the fallopian tube, uterus, or even epididymis, the validity of such measurements is questionable. Experiments with one sperm antigen, sperm-specific LDH-C4, with baboons (both male and female), in which some protection against pregnancy was achieved, there was no relationship between circulating antibody levels and fertility status (Mahony et al., 2000; O'Hern et al., 1995). In addition, a similar lack of correlation between antibody levels and fertility status has been seen in macaque monkeys (Tollner et al., 2002). In ongoing trials of sperm antigen vaccines, antibody levels will be measured in the female reproductive tract secretions, followed by fertility studies with monkeys after active immunization (primary injection with two boosts).

Some have also raised ethical considerations about contraceptive vaccines. For example, an anti-hCG vaccine would block the establishment of pregnancy after fertilization, and thus is viewed unfavorably by some as an abortifacient rather than a contraceptive. In addition, following the Indian clinical trial, some women's groups expressed concern that this method could be used to sterilize women without their knowledge or that it could be administered along with routine vaccinations without their knowledge. It is imperative that consumers be involved in the continuing development of such immunocontraceptives to provide knowledge and reassurance. Good science alone is not enough to ensure uptake of such a method. Creative introduction strategies will be critical to ensure the widespread acceptance of such new contraceptive methods once an effective and safe vaccine is obtained.

The lack of funding for translational research to move promising leads from proof of concept to a product is a major impediment, but the lack of papers on immunocontraception at annual meetings of major scientific societies also indicates a waning interest in the field. A helpful means of reenergizing the field would be the establishment of an annual immunocontraceptive workshop, modeled after the ovarian or testis workshops. NICHD could play a leading role in the organization and funding of such an undertaking.

REFERENCES

Aitken RJ. 2002. Immunocontraceptive vaccines for human use. *J Reprod Immunol* 57(1–2):273–287.

Amaral E, Faundes A, Zaneveld L, Waller D, Garg S. 1999. Study of the vaginal tolerance to Acidform, an acid-buffering, bioadhesive gel. *Contraception* 60(6):361–366.

Bebb RA, Anawalt BD, Christensen RB, Paulsen CA, Bremner WJ, Matsumoto AM. 1996. Combined administration of levonorgestrel and testosterone induces more rapid and effective suppression of spermatogenesis than testosterone alone: a promising male contraceptive approach. *J Clin Endocrinol Metab* 81(2):757–762.

Brown A, Cheng L, Lin S, Baird DT. 2002. Daily low-dose mifepristone has contraceptive potential by suppressing ovulation and menstruation: a double-blind randomized control trial of 2 and 5 mg per day for 120 days. *J Clin Endocrinol Metab* 87(1):63–70.

Cameron ST, Thong KJ, Baird DT. 1995. Effect of daily low dose mifepristone on the ovarian cycle and on dynamics of follicle growth. *Clin Endocrinol (Oxf)* 43(4):407–414.

Chen X, Xiao B. 1997. Effect of once weekly administration of mifepristone on ovarian function in normal women. *Contraception* 56(3):175–180.

Cheng CY, Silvestrini B, Grima J, Mo MY, Zhu LJ, Johansson E, Saso L, Leone MG, Palmery M, Mruk D. 2001. Two new male contraceptives exert their effects by depleting germ cells prematurely from the testis. *Biol Reprod* 65(2):449–461.

Cheng CY, Mo M, Grima J, Saso L, Tita B, Mruk D, Silvestrini B. 2002. Indazole carboxylic acids in male contraception. *Contraception* 65(4):265–268.

Chwalisz K, Brenner RM, Fuhrmann UU, Hess-Stumpp H, Elger W. 2000. Antiproliferative effects of progesterone antagonists and progesterone receptor modulators on the endometrium. *Steroids* 65(10–11):741–751.

Cook CE, Jump JM, Zhang P, Stephens JR, Lee YW, Fail PA, Anderson SA. 1997. Exceptionally potent antispermatogenic compounds from 8-halogenation of (4aRS,5SR,9bRS)-hexahydroindeno-[1,2-c]pyridines. *J Med Chem* 40(14):2111–2112.

Croxatto HB, Salvatierra AM, Croxatto HD, Fuentealba B. 1993. Effects of continuous treatment with low dose mifepristone throughout one menstrual cycle. *Hum Reprod* 8(2):201–207.

De Martino C, Malcorni W, Bellocci M, Floridi A, Marcante ML. 1981. Effects of AF 1312 TS and lonidamine on mammalian testis: a morphological study. *Chemotherapy (Basel)* 27 (suppl 2):27–42.

Fail PA, Anderson SA, Cook CE. 2000. 28-day toxicology test: indenopyridine RTI 4587-056 in male Sprague-Dawley rats. *Reprod Toxicol* 14(3):265–274.

Garg S, Anderson RA, Chany CJ II, Waller DP, Diao XH, Vermani K, Zaneveld LJ. 2001. Properties of a new acid-buffering bioadhesive vaginal formulation (ACIDFORM). *Contraception* 64(1):67–75.

Gatto MT, Tita B, Artico M, Saso L. 2002. Recent studies on lonidamine, the lead compound of the antispermatogenic indazol-carboxylic acids. *Contraception* 65(4):277–278.

Gemzell-Danielsson K, Swahn ML, Svalander P, Bygdeman M. 1993. Early luteal phase treatment with mifepristone (RU 486) for fertility regulation. *Hum Reprod* 8(6):870–873.

Gemzell-Danielsson K, Westlund P, Johannisson E, Swahn ML, Bygdeman M, Seppala M. 1996. Effect of low weekly doses of mifepristone on ovarian function and endometrial development. *Hum Reprod* 11(2):256–264.

Glasier A. 2002. New developments in contraceptive drugs for use by women. *Expert Opin Investig Drugs* 11(9):1239–1251.

Glasier AF, Anakwe R, Everington D, Martin CW, van der Spuy Z, Cheng L, Ho PC, Anderson RA. 2000. Would women trust their partners to use a male pill? *Hum Reprod* 15(3):646–649.

Global Microbicide Project. 2000. *Global Microbicide Project . . . Responding to an Urgent Need.* [Online]. Available: http://www.gmp.org/ [accessed August 2003].

Grima J, Silvestrini B, Cheng CY. 2001. Reversible inhibition of spermatogenesis in rats using a new male contraceptive, 1-(2,4-dichlorobenzyl)-indazole-3-carbohydrazide. *Biol Reprod* 64(5):1500–1508.

Gu YQ, Wang XH, Xu D, Peng L, Cheng LF, Huang MK, Huang ZJ, Zhang GY. 2003. A multicenter contraceptive efficacy study of injectable testosterone undecanoate in healthy Chinese men. *J Clin Endocrinol Metab* 88(2):562–568.

Gupta SK. 2003. Status of immunodiagnosis and immunocontraceptive vaccines in India. *Adv Biochem Eng Biotechnol* 85:181–214.

Hapangama DK, Brown A, Glasier AF, Baird DT. 2001. Feasibility of administering mifepristone as a once a month contraceptive pill. *Hum Reprod* 16(6):1145–1150.

Hodgen GD. 1991. Antiprogestins: the political chemistry of RU486. *Fertil Steril* 56(3):394–395.

Institute of Medicine. 1996. *Contraceptive Research and Development: Looking to the Future.* Harrison PF, Rosenfield A, eds. Washington, DC: National Academy Press.

International Partnership for Microbicides. 2002. *About IPM.* [Online]. Available: http://www.ipm-microbicides.org [accessed August 2003].

Kaisernetwork. August 21, 2003. *Daily HIV/AIDS Report, Science & Medicine FDA Panel Meets to Discuss Ways to Test Safety, Efficacy of Experimental Microbicides to Prevent HIV Transmission.* [Online]. Available: http://www.kaisernetwork.org/daily_reports/rep_index.cfm?hint=1&DR_ID=19464 [accessed August 2003].

Karolinska Symposia on Research Methods in Reproductive Endocrinology. 1974. *7th Symposium, Immunological Approaches to Fertility Control.* Diczfalusy E, ed. Stockholm, Sweden: Karolinska Institutet.

Kloosterboer HJ, Deckers GH, Schoonen WG. 1994. Pharmacology of two new very selective antiprogestagens: Org 31710 and Org 31806. *Hum Reprod* 9(suppl 1):47–52.

Ledger WL, Sweeting VM, Hillier H, Baird DT. 1992. Inhibition of ovulation by low-dose mifepristone (RU 486). *Hum Reprod* 7(7):945–950.

Mahony MC, Rice K, Goldberg E, Doncel G. 2000. Baboon spermatozoa-zona pellucida binding assay. *Contraception* 61(3):235–240.

Marions L, Danielsson KG, Swahn ML, Bygdeman M. 1998. Contraceptive efficacy of low doses of mifepristone. *Fertil Steril* 70(5):813–816.

Marions L, Viski S, Danielsson KG, Resch BA, Swahn ML, Bygdeman M, Kovacs L. 1999. Contraceptive efficacy of daily administration of 0.5 mg mifepristone. *Hum Reprod* 14(11):2788–2790.

Martin CW, Anderson RA, Cheng L, Ho PC, van der Spuy Z, Smith KB, Glasier AF, Everington D, Baird DT. 2000. Potential impact of hormonal male contraception: cross-cultural implications for development of novel preparations. *Hum Reprod* 15(3):637–645.

Massai R, Diaz S, Jackanicz T, Croxatto HB. 2000. Vaginal rings for contraception in lactating women. *Steroids* 65(10–11):703–707.

Meriggiola MC, Bremner WJ, Paulsen CA, Valdiserri A, Incorvaia L, Motta R, Pavani A, Capelli M , Flamigni C. 1996. A combined regimen of cyproterone acetate and testosterone enanthate as a potentially highly effective male contraceptive. *J Clin Endocrinol Metab* 81(8):3018–3023.

Meriggiola MC, Farley TM, Mbizvo MT. 2003. A review of androgen-progestin regimens for male contraception. *J Androl* 24(4):466–483.

Mishra PK, Manivannan B, Pathak N, Sriram S, Bhande SS, Panneerdoss S, Lohiya NK. 2003. Status of spermatogenesis and sperm parameters in langur monkeys following long-term vas occlusion with styrene maleic anhydride. *J Androl* 24(4):501–509.

Nieschlag E, Anderson RA, Apter D. 2002. Sixth Summit Meeting Consensus: recommendations for regulatory approval for hormonal male contraception. *Int J Androl* 25(6):375.

O'Hern PA, Bambra CS, Isahakia M, Goldberg E. 1995. Reversible contraception in female baboons immunized with a synthetic epitope of sperm-specific lactate dehydrogenase. *Biol Reprod* 52(2):331–339.

Passaro M, Piquion J, Mullen N, Sutherland D, Alexander NJ, Nieman L. 1997. Safety and luteal phase effects of the antiprogestin CDB2914 in normally cycling women. In: *Proceedings of the 79th meeting of the Endocrine Society.* Minneapolis: p. 227.

Silvestrini B. 1991. Lonidamine: an overview. *Semin Oncol* 18(2 suppl 4):2–6.

Silvestrini B, Palazzo G, De Gregorio M. 1984. Lonidamine and related compounds. *Prog Med Chem* 21:110–135.

Sivin I, Diaz S, Croxatto HB, Miranda P, Shaaban M, Sayed EH, Xiao B, Wu SC, Du M, Alvarez F, Brache V, Basnayake S, McCarthy T, Lacarra M, Mishell DR Jr, Koetsawang S, Stern J, Jackanicz T. 1997. Contraceptives for lactating women: a comparative trial of a progesterone-releasing vaginal ring and the copper T 380A IUD. *Contraception* 55(4):225–232.

Snow RC, Guzman Garcia S, Kureshy N, Sadana R, Singh S, Becerra Valdivia M, Lancaster S, Hoffman M, Aitken I. 1997. Attributes of contraceptive technology: women's preferences in seven countries. In: Sundari Ravindran TK, Berer M, Cottingham J, eds. *Beyond Acceptability: Users' Perspectives on Contraception*. London, UK: Reproductive Health Matters for the World Health Organization. Pp. 36–48.

Spitz IM, Croxatto HB, Robbins A. 1996. Antiprogestins: mechanism of action and contraceptive potential. *Annu Rev Pharmacol Toxicol* 36:47–81.

Stratton P, Hartog B, Hajizadeh N, Piquion J, Sutherland D, Merino M, Lee YJ, Nieman LK. 2000. A single mid-follicular dose of CDB-2914, a new antiprogestin, inhibits folliculogenesis and endometrial differentiation in normally cycling women. *Hum Reprod* 15(5):1092–1099.

Swerdloff RS, Bagatell CJ, Wang C, Anawalt BD, Berman N, Steiner B, Bremner WJ. 1998. Suppression of spermatogenesis in man induced by Nal-Glu gonadotropin releasing hormone antagonist and testosterone enanthate (TE) is maintained by TE alone. *J Clin Endocrinol Metab* 83(10):3527–3533.

Talwar GP, Singh O, Pal R, Chatterjee N, Sahai P, Dhall K, Kaur J, Das SK, Suri S, Buckshee K, et al. 1994. A vaccine that prevents pregnancy in women. *Proc Natl Acad Sci U S A* 91(18):8532–8536.

Task Force on Postovulatory Methods of Fertility Regulation. 1999. Comparison of three single doses of mifepristone as emergency contraception: a randomised trial. Task Force on Postovulatory Methods of Fertility Regulation. *Lancet* 353(9154):697–702.

Tollner TL, Overstreet JW, Branciforte D, Primakoff PD. 2002. Immunization of female cynomolgus macaques with a synthetic epitope of sperm-specific lactate dehydrogenase results in high antibody titers but does not reduce fertility. *Mol Reprod Dev* 62(2):257–264.

Trussell J, Vaughan B. 1999. Contraceptive failure, method-related discontinuation and resumption of use: results from the 1995 National Survey of Family Growth. *Fam Plann Perspect* 31(2):64–72, 93.

van der Spoel AC, Jeyakumar M, Butters TD, Charlton HM, Moore HD, Dwek RA, Platt FM. 2002. Reversible infertility in male mice after oral administration of alkylated imino sugars: a nonhormonal approach to male contraception. *Proc Natl Acad Sci U S A* 99(26):17173–17178.

Waites GM. 2003. Development of methods of male contraception: impact of the World Health Organization Task Force. *Fertil Steril* 80(1):1–15.

Weston GC, Schlipalius ML, Bhuinneain MN, Vollenhoven BJ. 2002. Will Australian men use male hormonal contraception? A survey of a postpartum population. *Med J Aust* 176(5):208–210.

World Health Organization. 1975. *Development of Vaccines for Fertility Regulation, WHO Sponsored Session of the Third International Symposium on Immunology of Reproduction, Varna*. Copenhagen: Sciptor.

World Health Organization Task Force on Methods for the Regulation of Male Fertility. 1990. Contraceptive efficacy of testosterone-induced azoospermia in normal men. *Lancet* 336(8721):955–959.

World Health Organization Task Force on Methods for the Regulation of Male Fertility. 1996. Contraceptive efficacy of testosterone-induced azoospermia and oligozoospermia in normal men. *Fertil Steril* 65(4):821–829.

APPENDIX B

Agendas and Participants in Committee Workshops

International Symposium on New Frontiers in Contraceptive Research
The National Academies
2101 Constitution Avenue
Washington, DC

TUESDAY, JULY 15, 2003

8:00 AM WELCOME REMARKS
Jerome Strauss, M.D., Ph.D., University of Pennsylvania

INTRODUCTION TO SYMPOSIUM
Allan Rosenfield, M.D., Columbia University

8:30 AM DISCOVERY APPROACH TO TARGET SELECTION AND VALIDATION
Moderator: Robert Braun, Ph.D., University of Washington
Moderator: Martin Matzuk, M.D., Ph.D., Baylor College of Medicine
Insights from the testicular transcriptome: Michael Griswold, Ph.D., Washington State University
Proteomics and the discovery of contraceptive drug and vaccine targets: John C. Herr, Ph.D., University of Virginia
Toward a comprehensive analysis of the genetic control of male fertility: Barbara Wakimoto, Ph.D., University of Washington

10:00 AM BREAK

10:15 AM Toward the genetics of mammalian reproduction: Induction and mapping of gametogenesis mutants in mice: John Schimenti, Ph.D., The Jackson Laboratory
Model organisms: The use of *Xenopus laevis* as a potential model for contraceptive research: Laurence D. Etkin, Ph.D., MD Anderson Cancer Center
Trapping participants of the oocyte-granulosa cell regulatory loop as potential contraceptive targets: John Eppig, Ph.D., The Jackson Laboratory

11:45 AM FROM TARGET SELECTION TO PRODUCT DEVELOPMENT
Moderator: Gregory S. Kopf, Ph.D., Wyeth Research
Charles Grudzinskas, Ph.D., Drug Development Consultant

12:15 PM LUNCH

1:15 PM FUNCTIONAL TARGETS FOR CONTRACEPTION
Moderator: Linda Giudice, M.D., Ph.D., Stanford University
Moderator: Gregory S. Kopf, Ph.D., Wyeth Research
Leptin peptide antagonists: Down-regulation of leptin actions in embryo implantation: Ruben Gonzalez, Ph.D., Boston Biomedical Research Institute
Gamete membrane fusion: A genetic approach: Diana Myles, Ph.D., University of California, Davis
Using chemical genetics to study regulators of fertility: Caroline Shamu, Ph.D., Harvard Medical School

2:45 PM BREAK

3:00 PM SMALL GROUP DISCUSSIONS
STD Prevention and Contraception: Should research be pursued jointly or separately?
Moderator: Nancy Padian, Ph.D., University of California, San Francisco
Target Selection: What criteria should be used to select promising targets?
Moderator: Jerome Strauss, M.D., Ph.D., University of Pennsylvania

Adoption of Contraceptives: What are the challenges associated with adopting contraceptives and how can they be overcome?
Moderator: Jacqueline Darroch, Ph.D., Alan Guttmacher Institute
Immunological Approaches and Contraceptive Research: What is the future outlook?
Moderator: Michael Harper, Ph.D., Sc.D., CONRAD
Evaluation of Contraceptives: What are the obstacles to preclinical evaluation and proof of concept in contraceptive development and how can they be overcome?
Moderators: Marlene Cohen, Ph.D., Independent Consultant; Ruth Merkatz, Ph.D., R.N., Pfizer

5:00 PM   ADJOURN

WEDNESDAY, JULY 16, 2003

8:00 AM   ADVANCES IN MATERIALS SCIENCE
Moderator: Lisa Brannon-Peppas, Ph.D., University of Texas, Austin
Overview of controlled release: Thomas Tice, Ph.D., Southern Research Institute
An overview of controlled release technology in contraceptive devices: Camilla Santos, Ph.D., Spherics, Inc.
Development of injectable, biodegradable microsphere products for sustained drug delivery: Mark Tracy, Ph.D., Alkermes, Inc.

9:30 AM   BREAK

9:45 AM   CASE STUDIES IN CONTRACEPTIVE DEVELOPMENT
Moderator: Anna Glasier, M.D., University of Edinburgh
Contraceptive microbicide development: Lessons from mucosal ecology: Kevin Whaley, Ph.D., Epicyte Pharmaceutical, Inc.; Johns Hopkins University; ReProtect, Inc.; Mapp Pharmaceutical, Inc.
Male hormonal contraception: William Bremner, M.D., Ph.D., University of Washington
Biosyn/C31G: Anne Marie Corner, M.B.A., Biosyn; Daniel Malamud, Ph.D., University of Pennsylvania; Kurt Barnhart, M.D., University of Pennsylvania

11:45 AM LUNCH

**12:45 PM CHALLENGES AND SOLUTIONS IN CONTRACEPTIVE
PRODUCT DEVELOPMENT AND EVALUATION**
Moderator: Regine Sitruk-Ware, M.D., Population Council
**Challenges and solutions in contraceptive product develop-
ment and evaluation: A U.S. regulatory perspective**: Lisa
Rarick, M.D.
Giving choices in family planning: Paul F.A. Van Look,
M.D., Ph.D., World Health Organization
**Applicability of contraceptive research to the need of
women in developing countries**: Ellen Elizabeth Hardy,
Ph.D., Universidade Estadul de Campinas, Brazil
**Exploring user issues that affect contraceptive development
and introduction**: Kim E. Dickson, M.D., Reproductive
Health Research Unit, South Africa

2:45 PM BREAK

3:00 PM PANEL DISCUSSION
Moderator: Nancy Padian, Ph.D., University of California,
San Francisco
Diana Blithe, Ph.D., National Institute of Child Health and
Human Development, National Institutes of Health
Laneta Dorflinger, Ph.D., Family Health International
Henry Gabelnick, Ph.D., CONRAD
Maurizio Macaluso, M.D., Dr.PH, Centers for Disease Control
and Prevention
Jeffrey Spieler, U.S. Agency for International Development

4:30 PM SUMMARY
Jerome Strauss, M.D., Ph.D., University of Pennsylvania

5:00 PM ADJOURN

WORKSHOP PARTICIPANTS

Nancy Alexander
Organon Pharmaceuticals USA
  Inc.

Amy Allina
National Women's Health
  Network

Suresh Arya
National Institutes of Health

**Kurt Barnhart
University of Pennsylvania

Wendy Barr
University of Pennsylvania

Margaret Battin
University of Utah

Gabriel Bialy
National Institute of Child Health
  and Human Development,
  National Institutes of Health

Holly Blanchard
Planned Parenthood of
  Metropolitan Washington, DC

**Diana Blithe
National Institute of Child Health
  and Human Development,
  National Institutes of Health

*Lisa Brannon-Peppas
The University of Texas at Austin

*Robert E. Braun
University of Washington

**William Bremner
University of Washington

Carolyn Brown
Private Practice-Physician
Arkansas

Stephanie Brown
Wyeth Pharmaceuticals

Erika Check
Nature

*Marlene L. Cohen
Creative Pharmacology Solutions,
  LLC

Doug Colvard
CONRAD Program

Carmela Cordero
EngenderHealth

**Anne Marie Corner
Biosyn

*Vanessa E. Cullins
Planned Parenthood Foundation
  of America

*Jacqueline E. Darroch
Alan Guttmacher Institute

Louis Depaolo
NICHD, NIH

---

*Committee Member
**Workshop Speaker
*** Sponsor Representative

**Kim E. Dickson
Reproductive Health Research
  Unit, South Africa

**Laneta Dorflinger
Family Health International

Regine Douthard
USAID

Allison Doyle
Johns Hopkins University

Charlotte Ellertson
Ibis Reproductive Health

Collette Eccleston
National Academy of Sciences

Eugenia Eckard
Office of Population Affairs

Edward Eddy
NIEHS, NIH

**John Eppig
The Jackson Laboratory

**Laurence D Etkin
MD Anderson Cancer Center

**Henry Gabelnick
CONRAD

**Ruben Gonzalez
Boston Biomedical Research
  Institute

**Mike Griswold
Washington State University

** Charles V. Grudzinskas
Drug Development Consultant

*Mahmoud Fathalla
Assiut University, Egypt

Mary Feeney
National Academy of Sciences

Shira Fischer
Institute of Medicine

Karin French
Takoma Park, MD

*Linda C. Giudice
Stanford University Medical
  Center

*Anna Glasier
Lothian Primary Care NHS Trust

Phyllis Greenberger
Society for Women's Health
  Research

Gary Grubb
Wyeth Research

**Ellen Elizabeth Hardy
Universidade Estadul de
  Campinas, Brazil

*Michael Harper
Eastern Virginia Medical School

Florence Haseltine
National Institute of Child Health
  and Human Development,
  National Institutes of Health

Joanne Hawana
The Blue Sheet

**John C. Herr
University of Virginia

Maria Herrero
University of Virginia

Laura Hessburg
National Family Planning and
    Reproductive Health
    Association

Mai Hijazi
USAID

Tom Hollon
The Scientist

Judith Johnson
Library of Congress

Michael Kafrissen
Ortho-McNeil Pharmaceutical

Mihira Karra
USAID

Sarah Kieweg
Duke University

Hyun K. Kim
National Institutes of Health

*Greg Kopf
Discovery Women's Health
    Research Institute, Wyeth
    Research

Trisha Lamphear
Alliance for Microbicide
    Development

June Lee
National Institutes of Health

Phyllis Leppert
National Institute of Child Health
    and Human Development,
    National Institutes of Health

Yi-Nan Lin
Baylor College of Medicine

Kim Lundberg
George Washington University

Joanne Luoto
National Institutes of Health

**Maurizio Macaluso
Centers for Disease Control and
    Prevention

Trent Mackay
CPR/NICHD/NIH

**Daniel Malamud
University of Pennsylvania

Judy Manning
U.S. Agency for International
    Development

Steve Marcus
Newton, MA

Danica Marinac-Dabic
Center for Devices and
    Radiological Health

---

*Committee Member
**Workshop Speaker
*** Sponsor Representative

*Martin Matzuk
Baylor College of Medicine

Elizabeth McCarthy
Institute of Medicine

Janice Mehler
The National Academies

*Ruth Merkatz
Pfizer, Inc.

Nigel Mcwilliam
CONRAD

Kate Miller
Ibis Reproductive Health

Marjorie Miller
Wyeth

Shirine Mohagheghpour
Planned Parenthood Federation
of America

Kirsten Moore
Reproductive Health
Technologies Project

Johanna Morfesis
Planned Parenthood Federation
of America, Inc

Tamarah Moss
Advocates for Youth

**Diana Myles
University of California, Davis

Sharyl Nass
Institute of Medicine

Deborah O'Brien
University of North Carolina
School of Medicine

Ann O'Hanlon
National Partnership for Women
& Families

*Nancy Padian
University of California, San
Francisco

***Gordon Perkin
Bill and Melinda Gates
Foundation

Tracy Rankin
National Institutes of Child
Health and Human
Development

**Lisa Rarick
Formerly, U.S. Food and Drug
Administration

Neelakanta Ravindranath
Georgetown University Medical
Center

Pat Reichelderfer
NICHD

Ericka Reid
National Academy of Engineering

**Allan Rosenfield
Columbia University

**Camilla Santos
Spherics, Inc.

Kate Schaffer
Ibis Reproductive Health

Gerald Schatten
Pittsburgh Development Center

**John Schimenti
The Jackson Laboratory

**Caroline Shamu
Harvard Medical School

Karen Shea
Planned Parenthood Federation
    of America

Emily Shen
Wyeth Pharmaceuticals

Wayne Shields
Association of Reproductive
    Health Professionals

Viviana Simon
Society for Women's Health
    Research

Ashley Simons-Rudolph
The George Washington
    University

*Regine Sitruk-Ware
Population Council

Harris Solomon
USAID

Jeff Solomon
Wyeth Pharmaceuticals

**Jeffrey Spieler
U.S. Agency for International
    Development

Robert Spirtas
National Institute of Child Health
    and Human Development,
    National Institutes of Health

Felicia Stewart
University of California, San
    Francisco

*Jerome Strauss III
University of Pennsylvania
    Medical Center

Gretchen Stuart
UT Southwestern Medical Center

Amy Swann
Association of Reproductive
    Health Professionals

Sheila Talafous
Wyeth Pharmaceuticals

Joseph Tash
University of Kansas Medical
    Center

John Townsend
Population Council

**Mark Tracy
Alkermes, Inc.

*Committee Member
**Workshop Speaker
*** Sponsor Representative

Theresa Van Der Vlugt
Food and Drug Administration

**Paul F.A. Van Look
World Health Organization

Ulyana Vjugiua
Johns Hopkins University

Kirsten Vogelsong
World Health Organization

**Barbara Wakimoto
University of Washington

Tracy Weitz
UCSF Center for Reproductive
  Health Research & Policy

**Kevin Whaley
Epicyte

Merrick Wright
Johns Hopkins School of Public
  Health

Wei Yan
Baylor College of Medicine

Koji Yoshinaga
NICHD, NIH

APPENDIX C

Committee Biographies

Jerome F. Strauss III, M.D., Ph.D., is the Luigi Mastroianni, Jr. Professor and director of the Center for Research on Reproduction and Women's Health at the University of Pennsylvania Medical Center, and associate chairman, Department of Obstetrics and Gynecology. Dr. Strauss's laboratory has three primary interests: (1) the regulation of steroid hormone synthesis in ovary and placenta, (2) polycystic ovary syndrome, (3) the biology of fetal membranes, and (4) the molecular basis of sperm motility. Dr. Strauss is a member of the Institute of Medicine, the National Advisory Child Health and Human Development Council, and is the current president of the Society for Gynecologic Investigation. He also serves as the U.S. chair of the Indo-U.S. Joint Working Group on Contraceptive Development and Reproductive Health.

Lisa Brannon-Peppas, Ph.D., is a research professor in the Department of Biomedical Engineering at the University of Texas, Austin. With degrees in chemical engineering, her research efforts focus on finding ways to expand the utility of biodegradable microparticles and nanoparticles to more effectively treat and prevent disease through the targeted delivery of drugs. Formerly, Dr. Brannon-Peppas was president and founder of Biogel Technology, Inc. (Indianapolis, IN). The company, created in 1991, was a research-driven enterprise that specialized in applying the technologies of polymer science to controlled delivery, separations, biomaterials, bioadhesives, and other areas. The company was active in research, development, and preparation of polymeric materials in biotechnology, bioengineering, medical sciences, and industrial pharmacy.

212

Robert E. Braun, Ph.D., is an associate professor in the Department of Genome Sciences at the University of Washington, Seattle. His laboratory studies a variety of topics related to mammalian germ cell differentiation. One focus of his work is to understand the mechanism and the importance of posttranscriptional gene regulation in germ cells. A second research interest is the mechanism of androgen regulation of mammalian spermatogenesis. A third area of interest is the genetic control of germ line stem cell self-renewal. Dr. Braun has served as a standing member on the Reproductive Biology Study Section of the National Institutes of Health (NIH) and an ad hoc member on several special study sections. He organized the NIH Workshop on New Approaches to Male Contraception as well as a Keystone Meeting on Germ Cell Differentiation and is currently on the editorial board of the *Biology of Reproduction*.

Marlene L. Cohen, Ph.D., is vice president of Creative Pharmacology Solutions LLC. She is also adjunct professor of pharmacology at the Indiana University School of Medicine. She recently retired as a Lilly Research Fellow from the Lilly Research Laboratories, Eli Lilly & Company, where she worked for more than 25 years in drug development and was involved in all stages of product development, from target validation to clinical testing. Her work at Lilly covered a broad array of targets, including anxiety, depression, migraines, and obesity. She holds more than 25 patents and has published more than 200 publications in peer-reviewed journals while at Lilly.

Vanessa E. Cullins, M.D., M.P.H., M.B.A., is vice president for medical affairs, Planned Parenthood Federation of America, Inc. (PPFA), New York, NY. In this capacity, she oversees clinical services, clinical business development, the PPFA Nurse Practitioners Program in Women's Health, the newly established PPFA Multi-Center Trial Network, and Affiliate Evaluation Department. Her administrative interests center around improving the quality of reproductive health service delivery through data analysis, interdisciplinary problem identification, problem solving, project planning, and project implementation. She currently serves on the New York State Department of Health Committee for the Care of Women with HIV Infection and is a member of the boards of directors of the Contraception Foundation and the Association of Reproductive Health Professionals.

Jacqueline E. Darroch, Ph.D., is senior vice president and vice president for science at The Alan Guttmacher Institute, New York, NY. She has expertise in demography and sociology, with a specialization in reproductive health behavior. She has a long-standing interest in sexual and reproductive health and rights, especially in relation to public policy and public education, including topics such as family planning, contraception, sexually transmitted diseases, and maternal health. She has also studied contraceptive service delivery and financing and method use effectiveness.

Mahmoud Fathalla, M.D., is the professor of obstetrics and gynecology and former dean of the Medical School at Assiut University, Egypt, and is current chairman of the World Health Organization (WHO) Global Advisory Committee on Health Research. Former positions include director of the United Nations Development Program/United Nations Population Fund/WHO/World Bank Special Programme of Research, Development and Research Training in Human Reproduction; senior adviser, Biomedical and Reproductive Health Research, the Rockefeller Foundation; president of the International Federation of Gynaecology and Obstetrics; and chairman of the International Medical Advisory Panel of the International Planned Parenthood Federation.

Linda C. Giudice, M.D., Ph.D., is the Stanley McCormick Memorial Professor of Obstetrics and Gynecology, chief of Reproductive Endocrinology and Infertility, and director of Women's Health at Stanford at the Stanford University Medical Center. Her scientific and clinical interests focus on women's reproductive health, with a major interest in disorders of ovulation, infertility, endometriosis, embryo implantation, in vitro fertilization, contraception, endometrial biology, and stem cell research. She is currently coordinating a collaborative National Institutes of Health consortium for the genome-wide investigation of gene expression in the human endometrium relative to fertility and endometriosis.

Anna Glasier, M.D., is the director, Family Planning & Well Women Services, Lothian Primary Care National Health Service Trust, Edinburgh, Scotland. She is also senior lecturer, University of Edinburgh Department of Obstetrics and Gynecology. Her clinical research has focused on hormonal interventions for contraception, with a particular focus on emergency contraception. She has served on many committees of the World Health Organization that deal with contraception and family planning. Noted publications include Contraception—Past and Future, which was published in *Nature Medicine* in 2002.

Michael Harper, Ph.D., Sc.D, M.B.A., is professor of obstetrics and gynecology, Eastern Virginia Medical School, director of the Consortium for Individual Collaboration in Contraceptive Research, and director of the Global Microbicide Project of CONRAD. CONRAD seeks to develop better, safer, and more acceptable methods of fertility regulation, with an emphasis on suitability for use in developing countries. Priority is given to moving promising lead compounds through phase I and II clinical trials. Dr. Harper's previous experience as technical officer at ICI Pharmaceuticals involved research on antihormonal agents for contraception and cancer therapy and the discovery of tamoxifen. Dr. Harper worked for the World Health Organization/Reproductive Health and Research program from 1972 to 1975 and has consulted for the World Health Organization, the U.S. Agency for International Development, the National Institute of Child Health and Human Development, the National Science Foundation, and the Andrew W. Mellon Foundation.

Gregory S. Kopf, Ph.D., is the assistant vice president for contraception, Women's Health Research Institute at Wyeth Research in Collegeville, PA, and adjunct professor of obstetrics and gynecology at the University of Pennsylvania School of Medicine. His academic research interests focused on signal transduction in gamete activation, fertilization, and preimplantation embryo development. At Wyeth, his group is mining genomic databases in search of potential novel targets for contraception and is also working with a number of academic scientists who are using new technologies to identify potential targets.

Martin M. Matzuk, M.D., Ph.D., is the Stuart A. Wallace Chair and professor of the Departments of Pathology, Molecular and Cellular Biology, and Molecular and Human Genetics at Baylor College of Medicine. His research focuses on generating and studying transgenic mice with impaired fertility and ovarian and testicular cancer with the goal of identifying and characterizing novel genes and pathways that are critical for reproduction and that thus represent targets for contraception in humans. He has received multiple honors, including awards from the Endocrine Society, the Society for the Study of Reproduction, and the American Society for Investigative Pathology. In 2001, he received a prestigious MERIT Award from the National Institutes of Health. Dr. Matzuk has published more than 160 papers and holds several patents for modified forms of reproduction-related hormones and transgenic models.

Ruth Merkatz, R.N., Ph.D., is Director, Team Leader for Women's Health, including the contraceptive product line, at Pfizer Inc. Previously, she was the first director of the Food and Drug Administration's (FDA's) Office of Women's Health, where she worked on regulation of breast implants, contraceptives, and other issues of particular importance to women, such as breast cancer, sexually transmitted diseases, and osteoporosis. She took the lead with FDA's Center for Drug Evaluation and

Research to change FDA policy to allow women of childbearing potential to participate in early-phase drug trials and to ensure sex and gender analyses as part of drug development. Before joining FDA, Dr. Merkatz served as assistant director of nursing and director of Clinical Programs for Women and Children at the Jack D. Weiler Hospital of the Albert Einstein College of Medicine (AECOM), Montefiore Medical Center. She holds an appointment as associate clinical professor of obstetrics, gynecology, and women's health at AECOM.

Nancy Padian, M.P.H., Ph.D., is professor of obstetrics, gynecology, and reproductive sciences at the University of California, San Francisco (UCSF), and the Department of Epidemiology and Biostatistics at UCSF and at the School of Public Health, University of California Berkeley. She is director of the UCSF Women's Global Health Institute and of international research at the UCSF AIDS Research Institute, as well as co-director of the Center for Reproductive Health Research and Policy. She also served as vice chair of the University of California Task Force on AIDS. Padian has served as principal investigator on numerous federally and privately funded research projects with high-risk populations. Her domestic research currently addresses adolescent reproductive health among teenagers in immigrant and minority communities. The major objective of her international research program is to reduce the risk of HIV infection among young women primarily through the use of female-controlled methods of prevention, such as microbicides or barrier contraceptives, and through the development of programs that foster economic independence and thus reduce reliance on male sexual partners. In collaboration with colleagues at the University of Zimbabwe (UZ) 8 years ago, she founded the UZ-UCSF Collaborative Research Program in Women's Health located in Zimbabwe, where she currently has eight research projects, and more recently she was awarded two grants on HIV prevention among women in India and one grant on HIV prevention among women in Mexico. Dr. Padian is a frequent participant in annual National Institutes of Health (NIH) Office of AIDS Research planning workshops and in 2003 was asked to chair the workshop on international research. She sits on the NIH AIDS Epidemiology Study Section and is an elected member to the American Epidemiology Society.

Regine L. Sitruk-Ware, M.D., is a reproductive endocrinologist and holds the position of executive director of product research and development at the Population Council's Center of Biomedical Research. She organizes preclinical research and clinical development of new molecules designed for reproductive health care in men and women suitable for use in developing countries. She is a program director for a cooperative contraceptive research center of the NICHD. Prior to joining the Council, Sitruk-Ware had successively an academic career and then a career in industry in research and development. She taught and conducted clinical research in reproductive endocrinology at the University of Paris for 10 years. She was a member of the International Committee for Contraceptive Research, which was established by the Population Council in 1970. She is a member of several national and international medical societies. Sitruk-Ware has written eight books and over 200 articles and reviews, mostly dealing with women's health care issues. She served as adviser on several ad hoc committees of the World Health Organization and the National Institutes of Health. She received her medical doctorate at the University of Paris and is currently an adjunct professor at Rockefeller University.

Glossary

Acrosome A membrane-bound compartment at the tip of the sperm that releases lytic, egg-penetrating enzymes.

Acrosome reaction Release of acrosomal enzymes.

Allele Any one of the alternative forms of a gene that occupy the same locus (location on the chromosome).

Amenorrhea The absence or suppression of menstruation. This state is normal before puberty, after menopause, and during pregnancy and lactation.

Androgen Generic term for an agent, usually a hormone (e.g., testosterone), that stimulates activity of the accessory male sex organs, encouraging development of male sex characteristics. Androgens are produced chiefly by the testes but also by the adrenal cortex and the ovary.

Antibody A protein produced by B lymphocytes in response to contact with an antigen from a foreign microorganism or molecular entity and triggered by T lymphocytes. Antibodies attach themselves to the foreign antigen, and to nothing else. This signals other elements of the immune system, including monocytes and macrophages, to destroy the invading organism.

Antigen Any substance capable, under appropriate conditions, of inducing a specific immune response when coming into contact with a lymphocyte or antibody.

Antiprogestins A substance that inhibits formation of progesterone, reduces its uptake by or effects on target organs, or interferes with its carriage or stability in the blood.

Antisense RNA A complementary strand of RNA that blocks the transcription of a naturally occurring (sense) messenger RNA molecule by binding to it.

Autocrine signaling Secretion of a substance, such as a growth factor, that stimulates the secretory cell itself.

Azoospermia Absence of living sperm in semen.

Barrier method A contraceptive method that establishes a physical or chemical barrier between the sperm and ovum, e.g., condom, diaphragm, foam, sponge, cervical cap. Some of the barrier contraceptives are used in conjunction with a spermicidal agent.

Bioavailability The degree to which a drug (or other substance) becomes available to the target tissue after administration.

Biotechnology The collection of industrial processes that involve the use of biological systems. For some industries, the processes involve the use of genetically engineered organisms.

Capacitation A process that takes place in the female reproductive tract by which sperm acquire the ability to fertilize an egg.

cDNA *see* Complementary DNA

cDNA subtraction hybridization methods A technique used to identify genes expressed differentially between two tissue samples. A large excess of mRNA from one sample is hybridized to cDNA from the other, and the double-stranded hybrids are removed by physical means. The remaining cDNAs are those that are not represented as RNA in the first sample and, thus, that are presumably expressed uniquely in the second sample. To improve specificity, the process is often repeated several times.

Cervical cap Small latex or plastic cap that covers the cervix. Users of this barrier method of birth control must spread spermicidal cream or jelly inside the cap.

Cervix Literally, "neck"; the constricted part of an organ; the cervix of the uterus is the lower and narrow end of the uterus that opens into the vagina. For pregnancy to occur, sperm must pass through the cervix into the uterus.

Chemotaxis The attraction or repulsion of a cell by a chemical gradient. Chemotaxis affects the direction of motion only.

Chorionic gonadotropin A glycoprotein produced by the primate placenta that plays a role in stimulating ovarian secretion of estrogen and progesterone during the first trimester of pregnancy.

Clinical testing Trials to determine the safety and efficacy of a drug or device in humans.

Complementary DNA (cDNA) DNA that is synthesized from a messenger RNA template by the enzyme reverse transcriptase. The single-stranded form of cDNA can be used as a probe to find a gene.

Conception Generally the beginning of pregnancy. Conception is usually equated with the fertilization of the ovum by the sperm, but is sometimes equated with the implantation of the fertilized ovum in the uterine lining.

Condom A cylindrical sheath of latex, polyurethane, or sheep intestine worn over the penis during intercourse as a barrier method of contraception and as a prophylactic against sexually transmitted disease. Some condoms contain a spermicide to kill sperm to decrease the risk of pregnancy should a condom break or should semen leak over the outer rim of the condom.

Contraception Anything that acts against conception, and therefore, anything that prevents the success of fertilization or implantation.

Contraceptive immunogen Any molecular entity meant to directly elicit an immune reaction for birth control.

Contraceptive prevalence rate The percentage of women currently using a contraceptive method.

Contraceptive vaccines Vaccines which induce an immune response against proteins specific to the reproductive process and therefore block fertility.

Cytokines Growth factors and immunoregulatory proteins such as interleukins that are secreted by cells and act as intercellular mediators. They differ from classical hormones in that they are produced by a number of tissue or cell types rather than by specialized glands. Cytokines generally act locally in a paracrine or autocrine rather than endocrine manner.

Developing country The World Bank defines a developing country as one a low- or middle-income country (less than $9,265 gross national income per capita in 1999) in which most people have a lower standard of living with access to fewer goods and services than do most people in high-income countries. There are currently about 125 developing countries with populations over 1 million; in 1997, their total population was more than 4.89 billion.

Diaphragm A soft, rubber, dome-shaped device worn over the cervix and used with spermicidal jelly or cream for contraception. Diaphragms are circular, shallow, rubber domes with a firm but flexible outer rim that fit between the posterior vaginal wall (posterior fornix) and the recess behind the pubic arch.

Dysmenorrhea Painful menstruation. Usually cramping lower abdominal pain. May be associated with low back pain, nausea, diarrhea, or upper thigh pain.

Efficacy The effectiveness of a form of contraception.

Egg An ovum; a female gamete; an oocyte; a female reproductive cell at any stage before fertilization.

Embryo In humans, the developing organism from about 2 weeks after fertilization to the end of the seventh or eighth week.

Endometrium The mucous inner lining of the uterus.

Enzyme A protein molecule produced by a living cell that catalyzes chemical reactions of other substances without itself being changed or destroyed.

Epididymis A coiled tubular structure where sperm cells mature and are nourished and which connects the testes to the vas deferens.

Epithelium A membranous cellular tissue that lines a surface, a tube, or a cavity of a body, serving to enclose and protect other parts of the body and to produce secretions and excretions.

Estrogen The primary female hormones; any natural or artificial substance that induces estrogenic activity, more specifically, the hormones estradiol and estrone produced by the ovary. Estrogens are produced chiefly by the ovary but also by the adrenal cortex, the testis, and the placenta.

Expressed sequence tag A short cDNA sequence that has a single occurrence in the human genome and whose location and base sequence are known.

Failure rate The number of pregnancies occurring per 100 users of contraception per year.

Family planning Programs or services to assist families to control the timing of reproduction through effective methods of birth control.

Fetus A developing unborn offspring. In humans, the fetal period last from after the seventh or eighth week postfertilization (the end of the embryonic period) until birth.

Follicle A small secretory sac or cavity. One type of follicle is an ovarian follicle which is a very small sac in the ovary in which an ovum matures and from which the egg is released.

Follicle stimulating hormone (FSH) Anterior pituitary hormone which stimulates the ovary to ripen egg follicles. FSH stimulates sperm production in the testes in males.

Forward genetic screens Also known as mutational screens, these screens identify a gene on the basis of a phenotype, for example, infertility, by inducing random mutations in an experimental cell or animal and then mapping and isolating the gene that causes the phenotype.

Functional genomics The study of the structure and function of all the genes in a genome.

Fusion proteins Proteins formed by the expression of a hybrid gene, which is formed by combining two separate gene sequences, through recombinant DNA technology.

Gamete Male or female reproductive cell (sperm or ovum) containing a haploid set of chromosomes (produced by meiosis).

Gene A complete chromosomal segment responsible for making a functional product, usually a protein.

Gene expression profiling Analysis of the products (usually mRNA) of all the genes expressed in a given cell or tissue.

Gene regulation The interactions between DNA and proteins that control the quantity and rate of the expression of a gene.

Genetic network A model of how genes influence each other, represented as a diagram with nodes and directed edges.

Genetic screens The process of testing individuals to determine whether they carry specific genes. See *forward genetic screens, reverse genetic screens.*

Genotype The genetic constitution of an organism or cell, separate from its expressed features or phenotype.

Germ cells The reproductive cells in the body; also called sex cells (in contrast to *somatic cells*).

Glycan structures A structure made of polysaccharides (carbohydrates that are made up of chains of simple sugars, monosaccharides).

Glycome A term designed to be parallel to the genome and the proteome, the whole set of glycans (polysaccharides) produced by an individual cell type or organism.

Glycoprotein A protein with covalently attached polysaccharide or sugar units.

Glycosylation The process of the addition of a polysaccharide to a polypeptide to make a glycoprotein.

Glycosylphosphatidylinositol (GPI) A lipid that attaches to a protein and is inserted into the lipid bilayer of the plasma membrane to anchor the protein on the surface of the cell.

Gonadotropin A substance having an affinity for, or stimulating effect on, the gonads, produced by the anterior pituitary or chorionic tissues of the early embryo.

Good Clinical Practice An international ethical and scientific quality standard for designing, conducting, recording, and reporting trials that involve human subjects. The International Conference on Harmonization (ICH) guidance provides a unified standard for the European Union, Japan, and the United States, developed with consideration of the standards of the rest of the world and of the World Health Organization. Ideally, compliance with GCP assures that the rights, safety, and well-being of trial subjects are protected and that the clinical trial data are credible.

Good Laboratory Practice A framework developed by the Organisation for Economic Co-operation and Development that covers the organization of test facilities and the conditions under which preclinical safety studies are executed, with the goal of generating only high quality and reliable test data.

Good Manufacturing Practice A set of principles and procedures which, when followed by manufacturers of therapeutic goods, helps ensure that the products manufactured will have the required quality. Various regulations and guides relating to GMP have been published by different countries and groups of countries. The United States has its standards monitored by the FDA.

Heterozygous Having two different alleles of a specific gene.

High-throughput methods Any approach using robotics, automated machines, and computers to process many samples at once.

Homologous Similar in sequence and function.

Homozygous Having two copies of the same allele of a specific gene.

Hormone A messenger molecule of the body that helps coordinate the actions of various tissues. Hormones produce a specific effect on the activity of cells remote from their point of origin.

Human chorionic gonadotropin (hCG) A glycoprotein hormone produced by the human placenta that maintains the corpus luteum and causes it to secrete estrogen and progesterone. Measured in urine and blood to detect pregnancy.

Human immunodeficiency virus (HIV) A virus that causes AIDS. It causes a defect in the body's immune system by invading and then multiplying within white blood cells.

Hypothalamus A part of the brain below the thalamus that helps to regulate basic functions such as sleep, appetite, body temperature, and fertility. It regulates the pituitary gland as well as other glands, including the ovaries and the thyroid.

Immunocontraceptive method Any contraceptive method based on interference of some step of the reproductive process by products of an immune reaction, be it antibodies or cells.

Immunogen Any substance that is capable of eliciting an immune response.

Implantation The process whereby an ovum burrows into the lining of the uterus 6 or 7 days after fertilization and attaches itself firmly. Successful implantation is essential to the development of the embryo.

In vitro Literally, "in glass"; a biologic or biochemical process outside a living organism.

In vivo Literally, "in life"; a biologic or biochemical process occurring within a living organism.

Infertility Failure, voluntary or involuntary, to produce offspring.

Injectable contraceptives Hormonal contraceptives given by injection. Two examples of injectable progestins are Depo-Provera (DMPA or depot medroxyprogesterone acetate), and norethindrone enanthate.

Interaction domains Small portions of proteins that mediate and regulate protein complex formation.

Intrauterine device (IUD) A flexible, usually plastic device inserted into the uterus to prevent pregnancy. May contain metal (generally copper) or hormones for added effectiveness. It produces a local sterile inflammatory response caused by the presence of a foreign body in the uterus which causes lysis of the blastocyst, and/or the prevention of implantation. IUDs may also prevent fertilization due to deleterious effects on spermatozoa as they pass through the uterus.

Ion channel A transmembrane protein that allows the passage of ions through a lipid bilayer down an electrochemical gradient.

Isoform Related but unique forms of a molecule.

Kinase A phosphokinase, an enzyme that catalyzes the addition of a phosphate group to another molecule.

Knockdown models Animal models in which the level of expression of a particular gene is reduced.

Knock-in models Animal models in which a specific gene has been added or overexpressed.

Knockout models Animal models in which a specific gene is deleted or rendered nonfunctional.

Lead compound A specific chemical that shows strong potential as a drug candidate to modulate a given target.

Ligand A molecule that binds to another; usually refers to a soluble molecule such as a hormone that binds to a receptor.

Lipidome A term is designed to be parallel to the genome or proteome, the collection of all the lipids produced by a cell or an organism.

Luteinizing hormone (LH) An anterior pituitary hormone that causes a follicle to release a ripened ovum and become a corpus luteum. In the male it stimulates testosterone production and the production of sperm cells.

Meiosis The specialized form of nuclear division in which the number of chromosomes is reduced to half by a second division in order to create sex cells.

Membrane protein A protein embedded in the membrane of a cell.

Menopause Cessation of menstruation; i.e., the last episode of physiologic uterine bleeding. After menopause, a woman is naturally infertile. Surgical menopause refers to the removal of a woman's ovaries before natural menopause occurs.

Method failure rates This measures the effectiveness of a form of contraception based on only the method itself, assuming perfect use. *See use effectiveness rates*

Microarrays A DNA microarray consists of a glass microscope slide or silicon chip onto whose surface thousands of specific DNA sequences are spotted. Incubation with a labeled sample of nucleic acid such as mRNA can reveal which of the genes represented on the array are expressed in the sample and their relative levels.

Microbicide An agent that kills or inactivates or prevents infection from various pathogens or microbes.

Monoclonal antibodies Identical antibodies—made from a single cell—that are generated in large quantities in the laboratory.

Monthly methods Contraceptive methods that only are used once each month.

Mutational screens Also known as forward genetic screens, these screens identify a gene on the basis of a phenotype, for example, infertility, by inducing random mutations in an experimental cell or animal and then mapping and isolating the gene that causes the phenotype.

Nucleotide A compound consisting of a ribose or deoxyribose sugar joined to a phosphate group and a purine or pyrimidine base. These compounds, including adenosine monophosphate, are the basic structural units of RNA and DNA.

Oocyte The developing female gamete before completion and release, known as ovulation.

Oral contraceptives (OC) Various progestin/estrogen or progestin compounds in tablet form taken by mouth; "the pill." Estrogenic and progestational agents have contraceptive effects by influencing normal patterns of ovulation, sperm or ovum transport, cervical mucus, implantation, or placental attachment.

Osteoporosis An abnormal softening, porousness, or reduction in the quantity of bone, resulting in structural fragility. Causes appear to include estrogen deficiency, prolonged immobilization, and adrenal hyperfunction, which result in more bone resorption than formation.

Ovaries The female gonads; glands where ova are formed; also the primary source of female hormones, estrogen and progesterone.

Oviduct The tube through which eggs travel from the ovary to the uterus.

Paracrine signaling Form of signaling in which the target cell is close to the cell that secretes a substance such as a growth factor.

Pathogen A microbe capable of causing disease.

Perfect use When the directions for use of a contraceptive method are followed and the method is used correctly for every act of intercourse.

Perimenopause Traditionally defined as the few (3 to 5) years surrounding a woman's last menstrual period; more recently it is being defined as beginning more than a decade before frank menopause, in the mid-thirties and early forties, coincident with the initiation of ovarian decline.

Periodic abstinence methods Contraceptive methods that rely on timing of intercourse to avoid the ovulatory phase of a woman's menstrual cycle; also called fertility awareness or natural family planning. 1. The basal body temperature (BBT) method uses daily temperature readings to identify the time of ovulation. 2. In the ovulation or Billings methods, women identify the relationships of changes in cervical mucus to fertile and infertile days. 3. The sympto-thermal method charts changes in temperature, cervical mucus, and other symptoms of ovulation (e.g., intermenstrual pain).

Periovulatory period The time period immediately surrounding ovulation when the egg is ripening and is released.

Pharmacokinetics The quantitative measure of drugs in the body, specifically, absorption, distribution, localization in tissues, biotransformation, and elimination.

Phenotype The characteristics of an organism under a particular set of environmental or ecological conditions, regardless of the genetic makeup (the genotype) of the organism.

Pituitary gland A small gland located at the base of the brain beneath the hypothalamus; serves as one of the chief regulators of body functions, including fertility. Most endocrine glands in the body are controlled by the pituitary. Also known as the hypophysis.

Polymer A macromolecule made of repeating (monomer) units.

Postmeiotic The stage after meiosis, when the number of chromosomes in the sexual cells has been reduced to create the mature form of the germ cells.

Postpartum After childbirth.

Pregnancy The interval from the completion of implantation of the blastocyst in the uterus until birth.

Progesterone A steroid hormone produced by the corpus luteum, adrenals, or placenta. It is responsible for changes in the uterine endometrium in the second half of the menstrual cycle that are preparatory for implantation of the fertilized ovum, development of maternal placenta after implantation, and development of mammary glands.

Prostaglandins A group of naturally occurring, chemically related long-chain fatty acids that have certain physiological effects, including stimulating contraction of uterine and other smooth muscles, lowering blood pressure, and affecting certain hormones. When prostaglandins are produced as the endometrial lining degenerates, they may cause mild to severe menstrual cramps, diarrhea, nausea, and vomiting. Oral contraceptives diminish the prostaglandins released by the endometrial lining, decreasing menstrual cramps in users.

Prostate A pale, firm, partly muscular, partly glandular body that surrounds the base of the male urethra in human and other mammals and discharges its secretion through ducts opening into the floor of the urethra.

Protein complex Structured ensembles of proteins and other molecules.

Proteome The entire protein complement of a cell or an organism.

Proteomics The science of defining and analyzing the entire protein complement (the proteome) involved in a particular biological process in a given cell, tissue, or organism.

Receptor A molecular structure within or on the surface of a cell characterized by selective binding of a specific substance and a specific physiologic effect accompanies the binding.

Recombinant DNA technology A series of procedures used to join together (recombine) DNA segments from different sources.

Recombinant proteins Proteins created by recombinant DNA technology.

Reverse genetic screens An experimental approach to find a gene's function by reducing its expression (via knockout or knockdown approaches) and then trying to identify the change in the phenotype.

Ribozymes Also called RNA enzymes, ribozymes are enzymes made of nucleic acids (RNA), not proteins, that can catalyze reactions, often the breakdown of other RNAs, and thus can be used to inhibit gene expression.

RNA interference (RNAi) An innate cellular process that is initiated when a double-stranded RNA molecule enters the cell, causing the activation of proteins that destroy both the invading RNA and the endogenous single-stranded RNAs with identical sequences inside the cell.

Sertoli cells Cells in the testis to which spermatids attach. They provide support and nourishment as the spermatids develop into spermatozoa.

Sexually transmitted infection (STI) Any infection that is communicated primarily or exclusively through intimate sexual contact. Sexually transmitted infections have been estimated to cause from 20 percent to 40 percent of infertility in the United States. STIs can adversely affect fertility by three primary mechanisms; pregnancy loss, prenatal deaths, and damage to male or female reproductive capacity.

Side effect An effect of a drug other than the one it was administered to evoke.

Somatic cells All the cells in the body besides germ cells; cells besides gametes and their precursors.

Sperm antigens Substances on or in the sperm that in certain circumstances elicit the production of antibodies.

Spermatozoon Male reproductive cell (pl. spermatozoa).

Spermatid Developing male germ cell that has not yet become a spermatozoan.

Spermatogenesis The formation of spermatozoa.

Spermicide A chemical substance that kills sperm, marketed in the form of foam, cream, jelly, film, and suppositories used for contraception. The spermicides used in almost all currently marketed spermicides are surfactants, which are surface-active compounds that destroy sperm cell membranes.

Spermiogenesis The part of spermatogenesis when immature spermatids become spermatozoa.

Sterilization A procedure that leaves the male or female incapable of reproduction. Sterilization is the most commonly employed method of birth control in the world.

Steroid hormone A group of related hormones (biochemical substances produced in one place in the body and affecting cells elsewhere), based on the cholesterol molecule. They control sex and growth characteristics. Testosterone, progesterone, and estrogen are steroid hormones.

Target A cellular structure or process that a drug or other therapeutic aims to modulate.

Testosterone Male sex hormone produced in the testes.

Transcriptome The complete pattern of gene transcription in a cell or tissue.

Transporter protein A protein that spans the cell membrane and carries specific nutrients, ions, and other substances across the membrane.

Transgenes Genes from another animal that are introduced into an organism by injecting them into newly fertilized eggs. The resulting animals are called "transgenic animals."

Translational research Research that aims to develop clinical applications of basic sciences discoveries.

Transposon A short sequence of DNA that can change location in the genome and normally contains genes that code for the proteins that enable it to change location.

Unintended pregnancy A pregnancy that was not wanted by the woman at the time conception occurred, irrespective of whether contraception was being used and whether or not a pregnancy was desired at some time in the future.

Use effectiveness rate or use failure rates This measures the effectiveness of a form of contraception, taking into account typical rather than perfect use. *See method failure rates.*

Uterus The hollow, pear-shaped, muscular, elastic reproductive organ where the embryo and then the fetus develops during pregnancy.

Vagina The 3- to 5-inch-long muscular tube leading from the external genitals of the female to the uterus.

Validation Verification that modulation of a target will produce, for contraceptive targets, a contraceptive effect.

Vas deferens The tube through which sperm pass from the epididymis to the ejaculatory duct and then into the urethra. It is this tube that is interrupted in the male sterilization procedure called vasectomy. Also called ductus deferens.

Vasectomy A surgical procedure in which segments of the vas deferens are removed and the ends tied to prevent passage of sperm. Vasectomy should be regarded as permanent, although reversal is possible in some cases.

Withdrawal (coitus interruptus) Removing the penis from the vagina just prior to ejaculation.

Zona pellucida The translucent, elastic, noncellular coating surrounding the ovum.

Zygote The fertilized egg before it starts to divide.

Acronyms

AIDS—Acquired Immune Deficiency Syndrome
AMPPA—Application of Molecular Pharmacology for Post-Testicular Activity

BLA—Biologics License Application

CDC—Center for Disease Control and Prevention
cDNA—complementary DNA
CICCR—Consortium for Industrial Collaboration in Contraceptive Research
CIR-LRP—Contraception and Infertility Loan Repayment Program

EM—Electron Microscopy
EST—Expressed Sequence Tag

FDA—Food and Drug Administration
FHI—Family Health International
FIC/NIEHS—Fogerty International Center / National Institute of Environment Health Services
FSH—follicle stimulating hormone

GATB—Global Alliance for TB Drug Development
GLP—Good Laboratory Practice
GMP—Global Microbicide Project
GMP—Good Manufacturing Practice
GnRH—gonadotropin releasing hormone

GPI—Glycosyl Phosphatidylinositol

hCG—human chorionic gonadotropin
HIV—Human Immuno-deficiency Virus
HPTN—HIV Prevention Trials Network
HTS—High Throughput Screening

ICCR—International Committee for Contraception Research
IND—Investigational New Drug
IOM—Institute of Medicine
IUD—Intrauterine Device

LCST—Lower Critical Solution Temperature
LNG-IUS—Levonorgestrel-releasing intra-uterine system
LH—luteinizing hormone

NCI—National Cancer Institute
NDA—New Drug Application
NICHD—National Institute of Child Health and Human Development
NIH—National Institutes of Health
NMR—Nuclear Magnetic Resonance

OR—Olfactory Receptor
ORF—Open Reading Frame

PQS—Protein Quaternary Structure

RAID—Rapid acess to intervention development
R·A·N·D—rapid access to NCI discovery resources
RNAi—RNA interference

SST—Signal Sequence Trap
STI—Sexually Transmitted Infection

UNFPA—United Nations Population Fund
USAID—United States Agency for International Development
USDA—United States Department of Agriculture

WHO—World Health Organization